Family Medicine in the Undergraduate Curriculum

It has been recognised by governments and healthcare organisations worldwide that for Universal Healthcare in pursuit of Health for All under the Sustainable Development Goals to be achieved, effective primary care that is integrated, accessible, and affordable for everyone is essential.

This practical guide is the first designed specifically to support those planning and conducting family medicine/primary care education within medical schools around the world. It offers medical educators a collection of concise easy to follow chapters, guiding the reader through the curriculum requirements with key references for further detail. Plain English and practical, deliverable advice, adaptable to different contexts, ensures the content is accessible to those educating medical students in any country, while the structure within sections ensures that family medicine doctors and educators can dip into chapters relevant to their roles, for example curriculum design for academic educators or teaching methods for those educating in clinical practice.

Key Features

- The first "how-to" guide dedicated to effective integration of family medicine teaching into medical school curricula
- Offers a strong evidence-based framework for integrating family medicine into medical schools
- Wide in scope, for academics and educationalists at all levels and in all geographies, reflecting and embracing the experience and variation in family medicine across the globe to produce pragmatic and effective information on which medical schools can base change
- Step-by-step introduction to the processes of literature review (establishing the existing knowledge base), choosing a topic, research questions, and methodology, conducting research, and disseminating results
- Supported by the WONCA Working Party on Education

The book is edited and authored by members of the World Organization of Family Doctors (WONCA) Working Party on Education, which is ideally placed to offer a strong platform for medical schools to integrate family medicine whatever the local context, enabling all future doctors, whatever their career aspiration, to understand the importance of family medicine to health systems and holistic medicine and encourage family medicine doctors to inspire students to consider a career in the field.

Series: WONCA Family Medicine

About the Series

The WONCA Family Medicine series is a collection of books written by world-wide experts and practitioners of family medicine, in collaboration with the World Organization of Family Doctors (WONCA).

WONCA is a not-for-profit organization and was founded in 1972 by member organisations in 18 countries. It now has 118 Member Organisations in 131 countries and territories with membership of about 500,000 family doctors and more than 90 per cent of the world's population.

Family Practice in the Eastern Mediterranean Region: Universal Health Coverage and Quality Primary Care
Hassan Salah, Michael Kidd

Primary Health Care Around the World: Recommendations for International Policy and Development
Chris van Weel, Amanda Howe

How To Do Primary Care Research
Felicity Goodyear-Smith, Bob Mash

Every Doctor: Healthier Doctors = Healthier Patients
Leanne Rowe, Michael Kidd

Family Medicine: The Classic Papers
Michael Kidd, Iona Heath, Amanda Howe

International Perspectives on Primary Care Research
Felicity Goodyear-Smith, Bob Mash

The Contribution of Family Medicine to Improving Health Systems: A Guidebook from the World Organization of Family Doctors
Michael Kidd

How To Do Primary Care Educational Research: A Practical Guide
Mehmet Akman, Valerie Wass, Felicity Goodyear-Smith

ICPC-3 International Classification of Primary Care
Kees van Boven and Huib Ten Napel

Family Medicine in the Undergraduate Curriculum: Preparing Medical Students to Work in Evolving Health Care Systems
Val Wass and Victor Ng

For more information about this series please visit: https://www.crcpress.com/WONCA-Family-Medicine/book-series/WONCA

Family Medicine in the Undergraduate Curriculum

Preparing medical students to work in evolving health care systems

Edited by

Val Wass OBE, FRCGP, FRCP, MHPE, PhD

Professor of Medical Education in Primary Care, Aberdeen University

Emeritus Professor of Medical Education, Faculty of Medicine &
  Health, Keele University, UK

Former Chair, WONCA Working Party on Education

Victor Ng MD, CCFP(EM), MHPE, FCFP, ICD.D

Assistant Dean, Schulich School of Medicine and Dentistry,
  Western University, Canada

Associate Director, The College of Family Physicians of Canada
  Chair, WONCA Working Party on Education

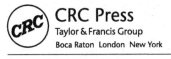

CRC Press
Taylor & Francis Group
Boca Raton London New York

CRC Press is an imprint of the
Taylor & Francis Group, an **informa** business

First edition published 2024
by CRC Press
6000 Broken Sound Parkway NW, Suite 300, Boca Raton, FL 33487-2742

and by CRC Press
4 Park Square, Milton Park, Abingdon, Oxon, OX14 4RN

CRC Press is an imprint of Taylor & Francis Group, LLC

ISBN: 9781032351858 (hbk)
ISBN: 9781032351841 (pbk)
ISBN: 9781003325734 (ebk)

DOI: 10.1201/9781003325734

Typeset in Bembo
by KnowledgeWorks Global Ltd.

Contents

Foreword   xiv

Preface   xv

Acknowledgements   xvii

Editors   xviii

Contributors   xix

Section I – Integrating FM into the UG curriculum:
Seizing the opportunity   **1**

1   Changing healthcare: Building the evidence for generalism   3
    C. Ruth Wilson and Shastri Motilal

    Introduction 3
    What is generalism? 3
    The relationship between generalism and family medicine 5
    Evolution of generalism 5
    Why is generalism necessary? 6
    Challenges of generalism 6
    The role of medical education 7
    Practical aspects of building the case for generalism: How to approach
      your dean 8
    Conclusion 8
    References 8

2   Defining family medicine   10
    Nagwa Nashat Hegazy and Anna Stavdal

    Introduction 10
    Defining family medicine: The terminology 11
    Principles of family medicine 11
    Global challenges 12
    The definition of family medicine 13

Role modelling FM values 14
Family medicine's role in society and health systems 15
Conclusion 15
References 16

3   Social accountability   17
     Maham Stanyon, Leilanie Nicodemus, and Robin Ramsay

     The need for social accountability in health professions education 17
     What is social accountability? 18
     Transferring socially accountable principles globally across
         healthcare systems 19
     Priorities for adapting social accountability to your context 20
     Conclusion 24
     Key documents 24
     Tools 24
     References 25

4   Developing an appropriate workforce for the future   27
     Archna Gupta and Raman Kumar

     Healthcare workforce 27
     The primary healthcare system and its workforce 28
     Primary care and its workforce 28
     Family medicine and its relationship to primary care and
         primary healthcare 29
     Supporting undergraduate family medicine training 30
     The importance of exposure to family medicine in
         medical schools 30
     Countries where FM is emerging 31
     Ensuring a sustainable workforce for the future 32
     References 33

5   Academic primary care: The importance of family medicine leaders and
     role models   35
     Chris van Weel and Ryuki Kassai

     Why academic family medicine is important 35
     A Japan case study 38
     Conclusion 41
     References 42

6   Barriers for change and how to overcome these   43
     Marietjie van Rooyen, Jannie Hugo, and Anselme Derese

     Introduction 43
     Influencing ministry and governing bodies on the importance
         of family medicine 44
     Working collaboratively with the health system
         (context of care) 45
     The role of the university and faculty in facilitating change 47

The medical school curriculum 48
The FM faculty and the students 49
Conclusion 50
References 50

7   Humanism in family medicine   52
     Martina Kelly and Chandramani Thuraisingham

     What is humanism? 52
     Why is humanism important? 54
     Why is humanism best acquired in family medicine in the undergraduate
          curriculum? 54
     Nurturing humanism in family medicine 54
     How is humanism currently understood in Asian medical schools? 55
     Conclusion 57
     References 58

Section II – What to aim for: Principles of curriculum design   **59**

8   Addressing population needs   61
     Hassan Salah, Saeed Soliman, and Marie Andrades

     Outlining the population needs of the country 61
     The need for community-oriented primary care physicians 62
     Population needs–based curricula: The role of PC education 63
     Exploring medical school undergraduate and postgraduate curricula
          for their responsiveness to community needs 63
     Addressing students' learning needs 64
     Faculty development 64
     Tips for incorporating population needs into the curriculum 66
     Conclusion 67
     References 67

9   Addressing patient and family needs   69
     Maria Sofia Cuba-Fuentes and Carmen Cabezas Escobar

     Introduction 69
     Learning to be person-centred 70
     Patient-centred clinical method 70
     Addressing illness, disease, and health 71
     Addressing families in the clinical encounter 72
     Shared decision-making 73
     Conclusion 74
     References 74

10   Competency-based curricula   76
     Maria Michelle Hubinette and Marcelo Garcia-Dieguez

     Defining competency-based education 76
     Competency-based curricula 77
     The added value of FM and generalism 79

Operationalising a family medicine competency-based curriculum 81
Conclusion 81
References 81

11   Designing an integrated curriculum   84
     Saima Iqbal and Val Wass

     Introduction 84
     The challenge of changing traditional medical education 85
     Curriculum integration 85
     What are the benefits of integrated learning? 89
     How to do it 89
     The family physician as a role model 90
     References 91

12   Values-based education: Integrating professionalism into the curriculum   92
     Kay Mohanna and Dinusha Perera

     Defining professionalism 92
     Defining values 93
     Nurturing professionalism 94
     Values-based practice 94
     Exploring global values 95
     Teaching professionalism 96
     Conclusion 97
     References 97

13   The formal, informal, and hidden curricula   98
     Hilary Neve and Richard Nduwayezu

     The formal curriculum 98
     The informal curriculum 100
     The hidden curriculum 101
     Addressing the informal and hidden curricula 103
     Conclusion 103
     References 104

Section III – Integrating FM into the curriculum: How to achieve this   105

14   Selecting for medical school entry: Nature or nurture?   107
     Sandra Nicholson and Tim J. Wilkinson

     Introduction and background 107
     Current challenges to medical school selection 108
     Ensuring best selection practice: What criteria should be used? 109
     Ensuring best selection practice: How should we assess? 110
     Ensuring best selection practice for FM values-based
          recruitment (VBR) 112
     Conclusion and areas for future research 113
     Five tips for global recruitment 113
     References 113

15   Early exposure to family medicine   115
      Victor Loh and Innocent Besigye

      Introduction 115
      Early family medicine exposure 116
      Socialisation of medical students 117
      Contextualisation of classroom learning 117
      Humanisation of medical care 118
      Implementing early FM exposure in medical school 119
      Conclusion 120
      References 120

16   Family medicine placements: Apprenticeship learning   122
      Elizabeth I. Lamb, Abdulaziz Al-Mahrezi, and Hugh Alberti

      Apprenticeship learning in FM 122
      Benefits of apprenticeship learning 123
      Challenges of apprenticeship learning 124
      Cognitive apprenticeship learning in FM placements 125
      Active learning in FM placements 126
      Role modelling 127
      Conclusion 128
      References 129

17   Longitudinal integrated clerkships   130
      Jill Konkin and Shrijana Shrestha

      What are longitudinal integrated clerkships? 130
      Establishing an LIC 133
      Enablers and challenges 133
      Conclusion: Why is this important for family medicine and primary care? 134
      References 135

18   Interprofessional learning   137
      Nynke Scherpbier and Carmen Ka Man Wong

      Defining interprofessional learning 137
      Challenges to interprofessional learning and collaborative practice 138
      Approaches to interprofessional learning 139
      Implementation and evaluation 140
      Change management 142
      Advocacy and leadership in family medicine 143
      Conclusion 143
      References 143

Section IV – Teaching and learning: Methodologies   **145**

19   Experiential learning for undergraduate medical students   147
      Thandaza Cyril Nkabinde and Julia Blitz

      Defining experiential learning 147
      Kolb's experiential learning theory 148

How can you encourage reflective practice? 148
Cultural humility: Orientating students to understand community culture 150
Active participation in learning: Communities of practice 151
Conclusion 153
References 154

20   Blended learning   155
     Pramendra Prasad Gupta and Deborah R. Erlich

     Defining blended learning 155
     What is the difference between "online" and "blended learning"? 156
     Types of blended learning 156
     Benefits and challenges of blended learning 157
     Guidelines for designing blended online courses: Ten tips 159
     Blending learning as we emerge from COVID-19 160
     Conclusion 161
     References 161

21   Clinical reasoning   163
     Simon Gay

     What can family medicine offer the development of clinical reasoning? 163
     Definitions of clinical reasoning 164
     What to prioritise for each learner? 165
     Application of best evidence 165
     Clinical reasoning development techniques 166
     Conclusion 169
     Acknowledgements 169
     References 169
     Other resources 170

22   Communication skills   171
     Mora Claramita and Jillian Benson

     Introduction 171
     The structure of the patient-centred communication style:
     The greet–invite–discuss 172
     The therapeutic relationship 174
     Multimorbidity 175
     Uncertainty 175
     The cultural influence within the FM context 176
     Conclusion 177
     References 178

23   Clinical and procedural skills   179
     Eric Wong and Krishna Suvarnabhumi

     What are clinical and procedural skills? 179
     Why teach clinical and procedural skills? 180
     What physical examination skills and procedural skills should we teach? 181

How to teach physical examination skills and procedural skills? 182
How to assess physical examination skills and procedural skills? 183
Conclusion 184
Teaching resources 184
References 184

24   Handling risk, uncertainty, and complexity   186
     Helen Reid, Jenny Johnston, and Amanda Barnard

     The challenge and opportunity of uncertainty 186
     Defining uncertainty 187
     Undifferentiated illness 189
     Complexity 189
     Risk 191
     Clinical courage 191
     Equipping FM learners to navigate risk and foster clinical courage 192
     Conclusion 193
     References 193

25   Well-being   195
     Pramendra Prasad Gupta and Shelly B. Rodrigues

     Defining the problem 195
     What is meant by well-being? 196
     Addressing well-being in undergraduate education 197
     Conclusion 200
     References 201

26   Supervision, mentorship, and coaching   202
     Oluseyi Akinola and David Keegan

     Definitions 202
     The roles 203
     Global differences 204
     Supervision: Setting up 205
     Supervising the learner at work: Directing and assessing activities 205
     Mentorship 206
     The benefits of mentorship 207
     Conclusion 209
     References 209

Section V – Assessment   **211**

27   Assessing clinical competency   213
     Mohamed Hany Shehata and Marwa Mostafa Ahmed

     Competency-based medical education 213
     Alignment of assessment with family medicine training 214
     Comprehensive competency-based assessment 215
     Assessing clinical competency 215

Mentoring and constructive feedback 217
Milestones and entrustable professional activities 218
Conclusion 218
References 219

28   The principles of feedback   221
      Chris Harrison and Hashmet Parveen

      Defining feedback 221
      The importance of observation 222
      Is there a magic formula to help you give feedback? 222
      Problems with feedback 223
      Avoid grades, be specific, and use narrative 224
      Avoid information overload 224
      Respect the individuality of the learner 225
      The importance of the learning environment 225
      Practical feedback tips 226
      Conclusion 227
      References 227

29   Principles of assessment and assessment tools   228
      Ching-wa Chung and Saniya Sabzwari

      Introduction 228
      The role of FM doctors 229
      Key concepts in assessment 229
      Reflective practice and constructive feedback 230
      Levels of competency 231
      Knows 231
      Knows how 232
      Shows how 232
      Does 234
      Barriers to involving FM doctors in assessment 235
      Conclusion 235
      References 236

30   Struggling students and fitness to practise   237
      Allyn Walsh and Zorayda Leopando

      The importance of assisting struggling medical students 237
      The multifaceted nature of medical student struggles 238
      Knowledge and skill deficits 238
      Professionalism and behavioural deficits 241
      Personal and health issues 241
      Multifaceted approach 242
      When remediation is insufficient 243
      Conclusion 244
      References 244

Section VI – Evaluating teaching and learning across the curriculum   **245**

31   Quality improvement and evaluation   247
      Esther M. Johnston and Akye Essuman

      Principles of programme evaluation and quality improvement 247
      Conducting programme evaluation 249
      Mechanisms for quality improvement 251
      Programme evaluation as a tool to ensure effective placement of FM
          in the undergraduate curriculum 252
      Conclusion 253
      References 253

32   Evidence-based practice: Medical education research   255
      Eliot Rees and Samar Abdelazim Ahmed

      Introduction 255
      What is research? 256
      Who needs research? 256
      Why produce research? 256
      Identifying a topic to research 257
      Constructing a research question 257
      Approaches to research 259
      Ethical approval 260
      Dissemination 261
      Conclusion 261
      References 261

33   Faculty development and continuous professional development   262
      Laura Goldman and Nguyễn Minh Tam

      Background 262
      Developing a faculty development programme for community tutors 263
      Needs assessment, goals, and outcomes 264
      Implementation 265
      Content 265
      Educational strategy 265
      Logistics 265
      Evaluation 266
      Key features of successful FD initiatives in family medicine 266
      Building an academic FM department through faculty development
          in a low-resource country 267
      References 268

Index   270

Foreword

Family Medicine in the Undergraduate Curriculum: Preparing Medical Students to Work in Evolving Health Care Systems is a much needed publication from the World Organization of Family Doctors (WONCA) Working Party on Education.

Editors, Prof Val Wass (UK) and Dr Victor Ng (Canada), as the Working Party's past chair and current chair, respectively, have brought together a diverse range of authors from 34 different countries to contribute their knowledge.

The book aims to offer a strong evidence-based framework for integrating the teaching of family medicine in medical schools. It will meet the needs of an international audience from a large variety of country contexts and address situations in high-, middle-, and low-income countries.

As early as Chapter 1, C. Ruth Wilson and Shastri Motilal write: "The remit of this book is not to simply promote generalism or create more generalists, but rather to highlight its place in medical education and healthcare delivery."

The 33 chapters ensure a comprehensive coverage of the topic and its many facets. It is comprehensive in addressing the integration of family medicine into the curriculum (Section III). However, the book also deals with important topics discussed worldwide such as faculty development (Chapter 33), assessment (Section V), workforce development (Chapter 4), and interprofessional learning (Chapter 18), to name but a few.

Undergraduate educators and family doctors, hoping to influence university curricula, will discover an informative reference book to refer to on many occasions, as they progress the various stages of integration of family medicine into undergraduate curricula. The book provides bureaucrats, university administrators, and faculty with a sound understanding of the importance of the teaching of family medicine to medical students and the importance of family doctors (GPs/family physicians) serving as faculty in universities, and teachers within their own clinics.

This book will contribute to improving health systems throughout the world by strengthening and guiding the teaching of family medicine at the undergraduate level. This in turn will no doubt improve health outcomes and better achieve "Health for All".

Associate Professor Karen M. Flegg
Australian National University Rural Clinical School
WONCA President-Elect

Preface

The Astana Declaration[1] in 2018 stated that, if Universal Health Care is to be achieved by 2030, strong primary care should underpin healthcare delivery across the world. Yet family medicine (FM) remains in various stages of development globally. The *Lancet* report[2] on "Health Professionals for a New Century" emphasises the need for education to adapt to produce an appropriate skill mix for changing healthcare needs. This means shifting the focus of training to ensure all future doctors have a balanced understanding of generalism and specialism. There is strong evidence to suggest that the more medical students are exposed to primary care, the more they consider a career in FM. Medical schools have a crucial role in preparing all graduates for evolving healthcare systems.

Yet medical schools globally have been slow to change. Undergraduate medical education remains secondary care dominated, and hospital focused. WONCA members have been asking how to bring the necessary change into their medical schools and how advice can be adapted to accommodate the significant differences in FM delivery across high- to low-income countries. Much of the published work is based on Western healthcare and medical education systems.

So, we decided to take up the challenge! The book aims to offer a strong evidence-based framework for integrating FM into medical schools whatever the local context and to enable all future doctors, whatever their career aspiration, to understand the importance of FM to health systems and holistic medicine. We felt we should embrace, not ignore, the experience and variation in FM across the globe. All chapters have at least two invited co-authors to include a high- and low-middle income country perspective.

We chose an approach relevant to both academic FM doctors involved in undergraduate curriculum development and FM doctors who teach medical students in their practices or would like to do so. The chapters guide the reader across the UG

---

1 Declaration of Astana. https://www.who.int/docs/default-source/primary-health/declaration/gcphc-declaration.pdf
2 Health professionals for a new century: transforming education to strengthen health systems in an interdependent world. https://www.thelancet.com/article/S0140-6736(10)61854-5/fulltext

curriculum, are short and easy to follow, and offer practical deliverable advice adaptable to different contexts. Key references have been selected for further detail.

One challenge was the global range in terminology for family medicine doctors and the need to distinguish between general practitioners (GPs) who in some countries are fully trained in FM but in others can become GPs with no training at all. Therefore, the term FM doctor is used consistently throughout the book.

We thank members of the WONCA education executive for their support and all the authors who worked so hard and enthusiastically to contribute.

Val Wass

Victor Ng

Acknowledgements

Our thanks to members of the WONCA Working Party in Education Executive for their support in the design and delivery of this book:

- **Marie Andrades** (Pakistan), South Asia
- **Carmen Elena Cabezas-Escobar** (Ecuador), Iberoamericana-CIMF
- **Nagwa Hegazy Nashat** (Egypt), East Mediterranean
- **Njeri Nyanja** (Kenya), Africa
- **Robin Ramsay** (UK), Europe
- **Chandramani Thuraisingham** (Malaysia), Asia Pacific

Editors

Val Wass throughout her UK career progressively combined clinical work as a family medicine doctor with medical education. The International Masters in Health Profession Education (MHPE) and PhD at Maastricht University built a strong platform for academic appointments in UK medical schools, including head of a new innovative medical school and editor of the journal *Education in Primary Care*. She has worked as a consultant in undergraduate and postgraduate education in over 45 countries, and her published research is widely cited. She holds several awards for an outstanding contribution to medical education, including the UK Royal College of General Practitioners' Williams Pickles and International President's medals, the Association for the Study of Medical Education's Gold Medal, and, in the 2015 UK New Year's Honours, an OBE.

Victor Ng is the Assistant Dean, Distributed Education and Associate Professor at the Schulich School of Medicine and Dentistry in Canada and a consultant physician in family and emergency medicine. He has held successive leadership positions in leading healthcare organisations and is currently Associate Director at the College of Family Physicians of Canada. He is Chair of the World Organization of Family Doctors (WONCA) Working Party on Education. Dr Ng completed his Master of Health Professions Education at Maastricht University and is a sought-after speaker on medical education globally. He has over 40 peer-reviewed publications and has sat on editorial boards of several influential international medical journals. He has been recognised for his contribution to medical education leadership and awarded the degree of fellowship by the College of Family Physicians of Canada.

Contributors

Marwa Mostafa Ahmed
Department of Family Medicine
Faculty of Medicine
Cairo University
Cairo, Egypt

Samar Abdelazim Ahmed
Dubai Medical College
   for Girls
Dubai, United Arab Emirates

Oluseyi Akinola
Department of Family Medicine
Cumming School of
   Medicine
University of Calgary
Calgary, Alberta, Canada

Abdulaziz Al-Mahrezi
Department of Family Medicine &
   Public Health
College of Medicine & Health
   Sciences
Sultan Qaboos University
Muscat, Sultanate of Oman

Hugh Alberti
School of Medicine
Newcastle University
Newcastle, UK

Marie Andrades
Institute of Family Medicine
Jinnah Sindh Medical
   University
Karachi, Pakistan

Amanda Barnard
School of Medicine and
   Psychology
College of Health & Medicine
The Australian National
   University
Acton, Australia

Jillian Benson
Department of General Practice
Adelaide Medical School
and
Faculty of Health and Medical
   Sciences
University of Adelaide
Adelaide, Australia

Innocent Besigye
Department of Family
   Medicine
School of Medicine
Makerere University Kampala
Kampala, Uganda

Julia Blitz
Department of Family Medicine
Centre for Health Professions
    Education
Stellenbosch University
Stellenbosch, South Africa

Ching-wa Chung
School of Medicine, Medical
    Sciences and Nutrition
University of Aberdeen
Aberdeen, Scotland, UK

Mora Claramita
Department of Medical Education &
    Bioethics
and
Department of Family &
    Community Medicine
Faculty of Medicine Public Health
    and Nursing
Universitas Gadjah Mada
Yogyakarta, Indonesia

Maria Sofia Cuba-Fuentes
Center for Research in
    Primary Care
Cayetano Heredia University
Lima, Peru

Anselme Derese
Department of Public Health and
    Primary Care
Ghent University
Ghent, Belgium

Deborah R. Erlich
Department of Family Medicine
Tufts University School of
    Medicine,
Boston, MA, USA

Carmen Cabezas Escobar
Medicine School
Pontifical Catholic University of
    Ecuador
Quito, Ecuador

Akye Essuman
Department of Internal Medicine
School of Medicine
University of Health and Allied
    Sciences
Ho, Volta Region, Ghana
and
Faculty of Family Medicine
Ghana College of Physicians and
    Surgeons
Accra, Ghana

Marcelo Garcia-Dieguez
Departamento de Ciencias de la Salud
Universidad Nacional del Sur
Bahia Blanca, Argentina

Simon Gay
School of Medicine
University of Leicester
Leicestershire, UK

Laura Goldman
Department of Family Medicine
Boston University Chobanian &
    Avedisian School of Medicine
Boston, MA, USA

Archna Gupta
Department of Family and
    Community Medicine
Unity Health Toronto
University of Toronto
Toronto, Canada

Pramendra Prasad Gupta
Department of General Practice and
    Emergency Medicine
B.P. Koirala Institute of Health Sciences
Sunsari, Nepal, India

Chris Harrison
University of Central Lancashire
    School of Medicine
University of Central
    Lancashire
Preston, Lancashire, UK

Nagwa Nashat Hegazy
Department of Family Medicine
Faculty of Medicine
Menoufia University
Cairo, Egypt

Maria Michelle Hubinette
Faculty of Medicine
Department of Family Practice
The University of British
    Columbia
Vancouver British Columbia,
    Canada

Jannie Hugo
Department of Family Medicine
University of Pretoria
Pretoria, South Africa

Saima Iqbal
Department of Family Medicine
Shifa College of Medicine
Shifa Tameer-e-Millat University
Islamabad, Pakistan

Esther M. Johnston
The Wright Center National Family
    Medicine Residency Programme
    at HealthPoint
Seattle, WA, USA
and
The A.T. Still University School of
    Osteopathic Medicine
Renton, WA, USA

Jenny Johnston
Centre for Medical Education
School of Medicine, Dentistry and
    Biomedical Science
Queen's University Belfast
Belfast, Northern Ireland, UK

Ryuki Kassai
Department of Community and
    Family Medicine
Fukushima Medical University
Fukushima, Japan

David Keegan
Department of Family Medicine
Cumming School of Medicine
University of Calgary
Calgary, Alberta, Canada

Martina Kelly
Department of Family Medicine
Cumming School of Medicine
University of Calgary
Calgary, Alberta, Canada

Jill Konkin
Faculty of Medicine & Dentistry
University of Alberta
Edmonton, Alberta, Canada

Raman Kumar
Institute of Family Medicine and
    Primary Care (iFMPC)
Greater Noida West, Gautam
    Buddha Nagar
Uttar Pradesh, India

Elizabeth I. Lamb
School of Medicine
Newcastle University
Newcastle, UK

Zorayda Leopando
Department of Family and
    Community Medicine
and
Department of Family Medicine
    and Community Health College
    of Medicine
College of Medicine
Our Lady of Fatima University
Manila, Philippines

Victor Loh
Department of Family Medicine
National University Health System
and
Yong Loo Lin School of Medicine
National University of Singapore
Singapore

Kay Mohanna
Three Counties Medical School
University of Worcester
Worcester, UK

Shastri Motilal
Unit of Public Health and Primary
    Care
Department of Paraclinical Sciences
University of the West Indies, St.
    Augustine Campus
Trinidad and Tobago, West Indies

Richard Nduwayezu
School of Medicine and Pharmacy
College of Medicine and Health
    Sciences
University of Rwanda
Kigali, Rwanda

Hilary Neve
University of Plymouth Peninsula
    Medical School
Plymouth, UK

Sandra Nicholson
Three Counties Medical School
University of Worcester
Worcester, UK

Leilanie Nicodemus
Department of Family and
    Community Medicine
University of the Philippines–
    Philippine General Hospital
Manila, Philippines

Thandaza Cyril Nkabinde
Department of Family Medicine
University of KwaZulu Natal
Durban, South Africa

Hashmet Parveen
PAPRSB Institute of Health
    Sciences
Brunei Darussalam

Dinusha Perera
Faculty of Medicine
University of Kelaniya
Kelaniya, Sri Lanka

Robin Ramsay
Usher Institute
University of Edinburgh
Edinburgh, Scotland, UK

Eliot Rees
Research Department of
    Primary Care and Population
    Health
University College London
London, UK
and
School of Medicine
Keele University
Newcastle under Lyme, UK

Helen Reid
Centre for Medical Education
School of Medicine, Dentistry and
    Biomedical Science
Queen's University Belfast
Belfast, Northern Ireland, UK

Shelly B. Rodrigues
Mosaica Solutions, LLC
Kansas City, MO, USA

Saniya Sabzwari
Department of Family
    Medicine
Aga Khan University
Karachi, Pakistan

Hassan Salah
Primary and Community Health
    Care
Department of UHC, Health
    Systems
World Health Organisation
Eastern Mediterranean
    Region

Nynke Scherpbier
Department of General Practice and
 Elderly Care Medicine
University of Groningen
Groningen, The Netherlands

Mohamed Hany Shehata
Department of Family and
 Community Medicine
College of Medicine and Medical
 Sciences
Arabian Gulf University
Manama, Bahrain

Shrijana Shrestha
Patan Academy of Health Sciences
Kathmandu, Nepal

Saeed Soliman
Department of Family Medicine
Cairo University
Cairo, Egypt
and
Primary and Community Health Care
Department of UHC, Health Systems
World Health Organisation
Eastern Mediterranean Region

Maham Stanyon
Centre for Medical Education and
 Professional Development
Department of Community and
 Family Medicine
Fukushima Medical University
Fukushima, Japan

Anna Stavdal
Department of General Practice
University of Oslo
Oslo, Norway

Krishna Suvarnabhumi
Department of Family and
 Preventive Medicine
Faculty of Medicine
Prince of Songkhla University
Hat Yai, Songkhla, Thailand

Nguyễn Minh Tam
Hue University of Medicine and
 Pharmacy
Hue Family Medicine Center
Hue, Vietnam

Chandramani Thuraisingham
Department of Family Medicine
International Medical University
Kuala Lumpur, Malaysia

Marietjie van Rooyen
Department Family Medicine
University of Pretoria
Pretoria, South Africa

Chris van Weel
Department Family Medicine/
 General Practice
Radboud University Nijmegen
Nijmegen, The Netherlands

Allyn Walsh
Department of Family
 Medicine
McMaster University
Hamilton, Ontario, Canada

Val Wass
General Practice and Community
 Medicine Team
The School of Medicine,
 Medical Sciences and
 Nutrition
University of Aberdeen
Aberdeen, Scotland, UK

Tim J. Wilkinson
Department of Medicine
University of Otago
Christchurch, New Zealand

C. Ruth Wilson
Department of Family
 Medicine
Queen's University
Kingston, Canada

Carmen Ka Man Wong
JC School of Public Health and
    Primary Care
and
Faculty of Medicine
The Chinese University of Hong Kong
Hong Kong SAR, China

Eric Wong
Department of Family Medicine
Schulich School of Medicine &
    Dentistry
Western University
London, Ontario, Canada

Integrating FM into the UG curriculum

Seizing the opportunity

Education is the most powerful weapon you can use to change the world.

Nelson Mandela

1

Changing healthcare

Building the evidence for generalism

C. Ruth Wilson and Shastri Motilal

SUMMARY OF KEY LEARNING POINTS

- Generalism is a broad-based discipline rooted in patient-centred care.
- Family medicine (FM) is the medical specialty that best aligns with generalist ideals.
- Over the years, generalism has evolved in keeping with patient needs.
- Evidence shows that generalism impacts positively on health at individual and population levels.
- Lack of exposure, low perceived status, and lack of pride are some of the barriers to generalism.
- The undergraduate curriculum must include generalism not merely to encourage more generalists than specialists but to ensure all students appreciate the needs and roles of both.

Introduction

Although family practice takes a generalist approach to patient care, generalism is not the priority of this group of physicians alone. All physicians, and their patients, will benefit from understanding the generalist approach to health. This chapter will provide a rationale for including generalism in the undergraduate medical curriculum and describe the contribution FM can make to a generalist curriculum.

What is generalism?

Persons seeking caring, curing, and healing will benefit from a skilled physician who will see them as a whole person, situated in their own family and community context. Family physicians would agree with the motto attributed to the Latin

DOI: 10.1201/9781003325734-2

scholar Terence, and revived by Maya Angelou, "I am human, and nothing human is alien to me".[1] For a physician, this orientation is displayed as curiosity to understand the influences on the health of persons and communities. This manifests in a broad range of competencies which are placed at the service of the patient. Generalism in medicine can be defined as "a broad-based discipline dedicated to contextualising care to the person and the person's social and physical environment".[2]

A generalist will have some knowledge of all the relevant factors affecting a patient, from the pathophysiology of various organ systems to the impact of the social determinants of health on a community's and an individual's well-being. The generalist may have skills or interests in several domains of knowledge, often generated by the needs of their patient population or community. A specialist, in contrast, may have some understanding of some areas of pathophysiology but will be expected to have an in-depth expertise in their own field. The key aspects of generalism are illustrated in Figure 1.1.[3]

> Generalism is a broad-based discipline dedicated to contextualising care to the person and the person's social and physical environment.

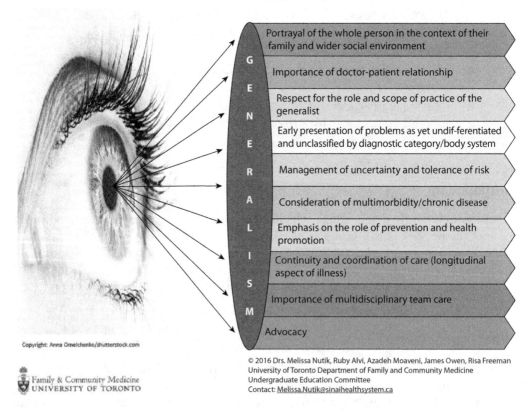

Portrayal of the whole person in the context of their family and wider social environment

Importance of doctor-patient relationship

Respect for the role and scope of practice of the generalist

Early presentation of problems as yet undif-ferentiated and unclassified by diagnostic category/body system

Management of uncertainty and tolerance of risk

Consideration of multimorbidity/chronic disease

Emphasis on the role of prevention and health promotion

Continuity and coordination of care (longitudinal aspect of illness)

Importance of multidisciplinary team care

Advocacy

Copyright: Anna Omelchenko/shutterstock.com

Family & Community Medicine
UNIVERSITY OF TORONTO

© 2016 Drs. Melissa Nutik, Ruby Alvi, Azadeh Moaveni, James Owen, Risa Freeman
University of Toronto Department of Family and Community Medicine
Undergraduate Education Committee
Contact: Melissa.Nutik@sinaihealthsystem.ca

FIGURE 1.1 Generalism framework: Key elements of medical generalism.

The relationship between generalism and family medicine

Several of the core values of family practice align perfectly with a generalist approach. Family physicians put the doctor–patient relationship at the centre of the care they give. Their commitment is to the person first before the diagnosis or problem may be evident.[4] Generalist physicians are equipped to provide care to all age groups, including the very start and end of life, birth, and death. This allows family physicians to be of value to communities, as their skills can adapt to the medical and health needs of their population and the community context in which they are situated. Family physicians can span the continuum of medicine, from prevention to curative medicine, rehabilitation, and palliative care. They provide a key link between population and public health, on the one hand, and primary and community care, on the other.

Along with this comprehensive set of skills, the hallmarks of FM are to be the first contact for patients and to offer continuity of care. Family physicians value communication skills and often have particular expertise in this area. These additional attributes are important for cost-effective person-centred primary care but are not synonymous with generalism. A generalist starts with the person seeking care by aiming to understand what they value in preserving their health, to learn about their illness experience, and to evaluate the limits of their knowledge. They can then advise or intervene and, if required, make effective use of specialists and their skills. This humane generalist approach is badly needed in medicine.

> Family medicine is the answer to the humanism that is needed in patient-centred care.

Evolution of generalism

Hippocrates (460–377 BC), who is considered the father of modern-day medicine, filled many roles as an astute physician with high ethical standards, an epidemiologist, a medical educator, and a scholar. Hippocrates' practice of medicine, at his time, therefore epitomised generalism. Until the 19th century, in America and Europe, the majority of medical practitioners were general practitioners practising medicine, surgery, and obstetrics.[5] While such practice may have been appropriate—given the knowledge, tools, and nature of diseases at that time—by the early 20th century, specialism had taken prominence. This was accompanied by a decline in generalists as lack of post-graduate training and the reduced prestige of general medicine gave way to other specialties.[6] The pendulum swung back in favour of generalism by the latter half of the 20th century as FM became a defined specialty. The factors that motivated these shifts were multiple, including the changing needs of the population, containment of rising healthcare costs, scientific advancements, and the move to consolidate general medicine as a specialty in its own right.[5]

> Generalism is not a new concept, but, over time, as medicine has adapted to the ever-changing needs of people, it has emerged as a specialty in its own right,

Why is generalism necessary?

Over the past century, there has been mounting evidence for the effectiveness of primary care. This has undoubtedly shaped healthcare delivery and population health. Research comparing primary with specialist care has shown that the generalist approach prevents illness and death and reduces health disparities in populations—all at reduced costs. Barbara Starfield (1932–2011) has been one of the most influential figures globally. Her numerous works demonstrate the value and need for strong primary healthcare.[7]

The statistics on population healthcare needs, first documented in 1961, revealed that one quarter of the population would consider consulting a physician at least once per month. This ecological study, when repeated 40 years later, showed that one-third of the community considered seeking medical care, and about 20% consulted a physician.[8] The relative stability of a population's medical needs over the decades is good justification for the generalist approach which focuses on the community level.

This chapter was written during the COVID-19 pandemic of 2020, a critical period in modern-day medicine which has tested the resilience of populations and health systems. All countries across the world have had to grapple with a challenging infectious disease and its related morbidity and mortality. Primary care medicine focuses on a patient's health. Public health, with its focus on population health, has never been so important. These two fields are complementary and lie within the generalist spectrum of primary healthcare. One key need, emerging from the pandemic, is to strengthen primary healthcare and build resilience globally[9] (Chapter 4).

> The COVID-19 pandemic has highlighted the importance of the complementary relationship between primary care and public health.

A generalist approach, though, in addition to its benefits at a population level, is important at an individual level. The concept of patient- or person-centred care has evolved over the past decades. The phrase, originally attributed to psychologist Carl Rogers, has evolved into a concept that encompasses understanding the patient's illness experience, building the doctor–patient relationship, and coordination within a framework of care.[10] These attributes resonate well with the generalist focus on the whole person and the environment in which they exist and seek medical care. When patient-centred care is applied, evidence shows positive outcomes especially on patient satisfaction and self-management.[11]

Challenges of generalism

Generalism has its detractors, particularly in a medical culture which holds the advances in specialty interventions in high regard. The saying "a jack of all trades and *master of none*" may be used to denigrate a generalist's skills. However, "a jack of all trades *is often better than a master of one*" also holds wisdom.

Generalism perhaps, at a glance, risks implying that generalist physicians can be all things to all people. This is clearly not possible. A generalist approach, at the level of individual patient care, will almost certainly require appropriate use of other skilled professionals. In primary care, the FM doctor works alongside other healthcare professionals; nursing being the key partnering discipline. Other potential primary care team members include pharmacists, social workers, physiotherapists, occupational therapists, mental health counsellors, and administrative support. Generalists also collaborate with specialty colleagues to address patient needs beyond their scope.[12]

> To deliver generalist care appropriately, a FM doctor must work alongside other healthcare professionals and collaborate with specialist colleagues.

Conversely, inappropriate use of specialists may lead to poorer outcomes, potentially at greater cost. This may be due to blindness to conditions outside the specialist's area of knowledge, over-medicalisation of self-limited problems, and ignoring preventive and lifestyle management options which could benefit the patient. Additional challenges to generalism include poor continuity and access to care, low status and lack of pride felt by those in the field, and gaps in competencies expected for comprehensive care.[13]

The role of medical education

Fortunately, some of these challenges are amenable to education. The remit of this book is not to simply promote generalism or create more generalists, but rather to highlight its place in medical education and healthcare delivery. There is a distinction between being a generalist and using generalist skills.[14] Medical school is an ideal place to gain an appreciation of, and learn, both. Generalists and specialists should be seen on a spectrum as opposed to a dichotomy, with both working together for the ultimate benefit of the patient.

Future doctors as part of their training should learn about generalism, both as a philosophy of care and as a specialty. Exposure to the theories underpinning generalism is important. The basic tenets of primary care, primary healthcare, patient-centred care, and the social determinants of health, must be taught throughout the undergraduate curriculum. This will help all aspiring physicians to better understand their role and what patients, irrespective of their pathology, want from them.

Promotion of generalism in the context of FM as a specialty has become mandatory in medical education. A systematic review of generalist placements during medical school highlighted that students on pre-clerkship FM placements were more likely to enter FM careers[15] (Chapter 15). Nothing can substitute for seeing consultations with real patients being role modelled by a primary care doctor (Chapter 16). Such rich learning experiences are crucial for all doctors in training. For settings that require completion of an internship after graduation, inclusion of a primary care posting during this period is key.

Primary care representation at career days offers another important strategy. This ensures students gain an appreciation of generalists' work, and do not view them as inferior to other specialties. Gaining insight into other practical aspects of generalism such as inter-specialty collaboration, patient-centred communication, and multi-professional teamwork is beneficial. Exposing medical students to generalism-in-action early and throughout the curriculum fosters broader perspectives and can encourage physicians to ascend into equally important roles of leadership, health administration, and patient advocacy.

All medical students should graduate with generalist skills whatever their future career pathway.

Practical aspects of building the case for generalism: How to approach your dean

- The need for medical schools to be socially accountable and educate physicians for the population they ultimately serve (Chapter 3)

- The benefit of undergraduates becoming well-trained pluripotent generalists prepared to undertake any residency

- The humanistic case for an education in person-centred generalist medicine as opposed to a technician's training (Chapter 7)

- The demands and opportunities within institutional resource allocation—how and when are students taught about and exposed clinically to generalist approaches?

- Monitoring of generalist content in curricular materials using validated evaluation tools[3]

Conclusion

A healthcare system where generalists and specialists are appropriately balanced, and work in collaboration with other health disciplines, is the most cost-efficient way to produce the best health outcomes. Every individual and family deserve to have a generalist clinician as their first point of access to healthcare and as a companion throughout their life course. Medical education, in the form of academic FM (Chapter 5), is key to the implementation of generalism.

References

1. Lencha S. Dr. Maya Angelou—I am human [Internet]. 2013 Available from: https://www.youtube.com/watch?v=ePodNjrVSsk (Accessed 13 December 2021).
2. Lee K.-H. A historical perspective of the barriers to generalism. Aust Fam Physician. 2015;44(3):154–58.

3. Nutik M, Woods NN, Moaveni A, Owen J, Gleberzon J, Alvi R, et al. Assessing undergraduate medical education through a generalist lens. Can Fam Physician. 2021;67(5):357–63.

4. Four Principles of Family Medicine [Internet]. Dalhousie University. Available from: https://medicine.dal.ca/departments/department-sites/family/faculty-staff-resources/preceptor-resources/principles.html (Accessed 13 December 2021).

5. History of Family Medicine over the Past 50 Years. Global and European Perspectives (AMF) No todo es clínica [Internet]. Available from: https://amf-semfyc.com/web/article_ver.php?id=2232 (Accessed 24 November 2021).

6. Flexner A. Medical education in the United States and Canada: From the Carnegie Foundation for the Advancement of Teaching, Bulletin Number Four, 1910. Bull World Health Organ. 2002;80(7):594–602.

7. Global Family Doctor: WONCA Online. The Barbara Starfield Collection. Available from: https://www.globalfamilydoctor.com/internationalissues/barbarastarfield.aspx (Accessed 26 November 2021).

8. Green LA, Fryer GE, Yawn BP, Lanier D, Dovey SM. The ecology of medical care revisited. N Engl J Med. 2001;344(26):2021–25.

9. Strengthening the frontline: How primary health care helps health systems adapt during the COVID 19 pandemic [Internet]. Available from: https://www.oecd.org/coronavirus/policy-responses/strengthening-the-frontline-how-primary-health-care-helps-health-systems-adapt-during-the-covid-19-pandemic-9a5ae6da/ (Accessed 13 December 2021).

10. Langberg EM, Dyhr L, Davidsen AS. Development of the concept of patient-centredness: A systematic review. Patient Educ Couns. 2019;102(7):1228–36.

11. Rathert C, Wyrwich MD, Boren SA. Patient-centered care and outcomes: A systematic review of the literature. Med Care Res Rev. 2013;70(4):351–79.

12. Stange KC, Ferrer RL. The paradox of primary care. Ann Fam Med. 2009;7(4):293–99.

13. Guiding Patients through Complexity: The Health Foundation [Internet]. Available from: https://www.health.org.uk/publications/guiding-patients-through-complexity-modern-medical-generalism (Accessed 27 November 2021).

14. Howe A. What's special about medical generalism? The RCGP's response to the independent Commission on Generalism. Br J Gen Pract. 2012;62(600):342–43.

15. Shah A, Gasner A, Bracken K, Scott I, Kelly MA, Palombo A. Early generalist placements are associated with family medicine career choice: A systematic review and meta-analysis. Med Educ. 2021;55(11):1242–52.

Defining family medicine

Nagwa Nashat Hegazy and Anna Stavdal

SUMMARY OF KEY LEARNING POINTS

- Family medicine (FM) has emerged globally as a clinical specialty and research-based academic discipline.
- The FM curriculum takes a holistic view of caring for patients within their community based on evidence from the natural sciences and the humanities.
- FM principles and core values are well defined. Regular revision to keep abreast of changing population needs and sociodemographics is essential.
- The WONCA (World Organization of Family Medicine Doctors) Europe 2011 definition of the core competencies and characteristics of FM provides a strong framework for teaching medical students.
- Family physicians can effectively role model patient-centred care and its professional values to students—a crucial prerequisite for the effective advocacy of FM.
- Trained generalist FM physicians are key members of the primary care teams essential to delivering sustainable healthcare systems and achieving Universal Health Care (UHC).

Introduction

Historically, FM is the modern, continuing representation of the original traditional medical practitioner, first referred to as a "general practitioner", by the *Lancet* in 1823.[1] The first doctors were generalists. For hundreds of years, generalists offered basic comprehensive medical care for diagnosing all diseases and illnesses, offering treatments which included surgery and obstetrics.

As medical knowledge developed, and technology evolved, many physicians chose to limit their professional activity to specific, defined areas of medicine. This era of specialisation started to emerge in the 1940s. During the two following decades,

DOI: 10.1201/9781003325734-3

the number of specialists and subspecialists expanded at an astounding rate, while the number of generalists decreased substantially.

As the age of specialisation peaked, a need for generalists with well-defined roles and skills reappeared. Globally, FM has emerged as a recognised clinical specialty and academic discipline with its own distinct curriculum and research evidence base drawn from the natural sciences and the humanities.[2]

In the United States, the American Academy of Family Physicians was founded in 1947. In the 1950s and 1960s, several colleges and academies of general practice and FM were established in a number of countries, including the United Kingdom, Canada, and the Netherlands. In 1972, WONCA was founded.

> Family medicine has emerged over time as a distinct specialty with its own curriculum based on the basic sciences and the humanities.

Defining family medicine: The terminology

When seeking to define FM, the international terminology can be confusing and used in conflicting ways.[3] It is important to distinguish between primary healthcare (PHC), an "organisational concept relating to the place, management, and work-load at the first (primary) level of health care",[3] and FM/general practice. These latter two terms relate to the work of the FM doctor per se and have been adopted and used interchangeably by WONCA. The term "GP" in some countries, though, refers to a general practitioner who has completed training as an FM specialist. In others, doctors can become GPs immediately on leaving medical school without training. The term FM doctor/specialist is only applied to those who have under-gone formal training. For the purpose of this book (see preface), to avoid confusion, FM is the term of choice.

> FM emphasises the generalist patient-centred relationship seeing the person holistically, in the context of their family and community, and delivered by doctors trained in the specialty.

Principles of family medicine

Ian McWhinney, long regarded as the father of FM, is credited with defining nine principles that underlie the practice of the family doctor.[4]

These are as follows:[4]

1. Never-ending commitment towards patients

2. Understanding the context of illness

3. Using every patient contact as an opportunity for disease prevention

4. Viewing a family practice as serving a population at risk

5. Developing a community-wide network of health and support agencies

6. Understanding the "habitat" of patients (even if they do not live there)

7. Caring for patients in office, home, and hospital

8. Acknowledging the subjective aspects of medicine

9. Being aware of the need to manage resources

These principles arose from the need to shed light on the important roles of family physicians and public education campaigns.[5] The concepts have now acquired even more relevance in a world that increasingly depersonalises patient care. Since then, the College of Family Physicians of Canada (CFPC) has condensed them into four principles on which to base the definition of a FM doctor[6,7] (Box 2.1).

> FM as a community-based discipline enables medical students to understand how a skilled family physician contributes to holistic patient care humanely in a defined population.

Global challenges

These basic principles remain important. However, as population needs change worldwide, the role of FM in healthcare systems faces many different challenges.[7] With escalating migration, there is increasing patient cultural diversity in contrast to the relative homogeneity of the past. This can create difficult ethical dilemmas. Ageing has impacted on disease profiles and service delivery. Family structures and patient expectations have changed and placed different demands on treatment and prevention. In some countries, FM is delivered from secondary care centres. Not all FM doctors deliver all services; maternity care and paediatrics may remain the remit of secondary care specialists.

This fragmentation has placed pressure on continuity of care—a core value many seek to preserve.[8] Thus, although in 2001 the Norwegian College of General Practice originally launched their statement identifying the seven theses, "Sju teser", on the principles, purposes, and core values of FM, these were

---

BOX 2.1 FOUR PRINCIPLES FOR FAMILY MEDICINE: COLLEGE OF FAMILY PHYSICIANS OF CANADA[8]

1. The doctor–patient relationship is central to the role of the family physician.
2. The family physician must be a skilled clinician.
3. Family medicine is a community-based discipline.
4. The family physician is a resource to a defined patient population.

subsequently modified in 2021.[8] This illustrates how healthcare is constantly changing and constant revision of specialty core values is needed. It is important that medical students understand these relationships. Globally too, wide variance in sociodemographics inevitably means that values need to be defined regionally. For example, in the African context, family physicians developed a list of 29 core values and prioritised 5—collaborative care, comprehensive care, continuity of care, lifelong learning, and patient–centred care.[9]

> Medical students should understand how changing population needs and sociodemography impact on the core values of family practice.

The definition of family medicine

It is not surprising that globally there are many different ways in which FM is defined. The definition we choose to use is that adopted by WONCA Europe as published in 2011[10] (Box 2.2). It comprehensively encapsulates the generalist principles underpinning the specialty and provides a strong framework on which to base undergraduate teaching.

Originally published in 2002, after an extensive and broad brainstorm process in the European FM community, the 2011 definition has been captured visually in the "WONCA Tree"[10] (Figure 2.1). This is useful for illustrating the daily work of the family doctor, teaching, and advocacy. It beautifully highlights for medical students the essential concepts, core professional competencies, and approaches to learning FM.

BOX 2.2 THE WONCA EUROPE DEFINITION OF FAMILY MEDICINE 1991[11]

"The general practitioner or family physician is the physician who is primarily responsible for providing comprehensive care to every individual seeking medical care and arranging for other health personnel to provide services when necessary. The general practitioner/family physician functions as a generalist who accepts everyone seeking care, whereas other health providers limit access to their services based on age, sex or diagnosis. The general practitioner/family physician cares for the individual in the context of the family, and the family in the context of the community, irrespective of race, religion, culture or social class. He is clinically competent to provide the greater part of their care after considering their cultural, socio-economic, and psychological background. In addition, he takes personal responsibility for providing comprehensive and continuing care for his patients. The general practitioner/family physician exercises his/her professional role by providing care, either directly or through the services of others according to their health needs and resources available within the community he/she serves."

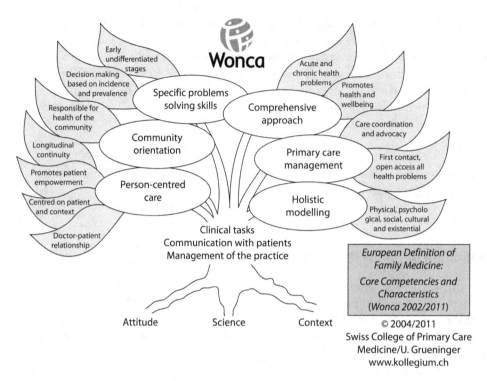

FIGURE 2.1 The Wonca Tree.[10]

Defining and operationalising the core values and principles for FM is an ongoing process.

Role modelling FM values

The drive to maintain the essence of FM as set out by McWhinney,[3] in the face of the concerns about the fragmentation described above, has led to ongoing debate and emerging evidence on FM values, which medical students need to witness and understand. These values include patient-centred care, the continuity of the patient–doctor relationship, the role of the doctor as a collaborator, the promotion of equity of care, and demonstrating the professional values underpinning FM practice.

As continuity of care is appreciated by patients, it creates trust in the doctor–patient relationship and further supports patient-centredness which has been shown to improve healthcare outcomes.[11] Repeated contact over time earns trust—a process FM doctors can role model to medical students. Similarly, patient presentations and symptoms that initially appear to be independent of each other can be shown to relate holistically to each other within the context of the family and the community.

The WONCA tree (Figure 2.1) can be used to demonstrate how a patient's experience of illness includes their feelings about being ill, their ideas about what is wrong with them, the impact of the symptoms on their daily functioning, and their expectations of what should be done. Similarly, role modelling collaborative practice within the multi-professional primary care team, and the quality of care received by patients each time they engage with the primary healthcare system, is essential.[12,13] Family physicians can demonstrate how equitable standards of healthcare must be tailored to the community context. Role modelling professionalism in practice highlights that family physicians remain committed to education, research, and quality development.

> Professionally role modelling to medical students of the values underpinning FM is essential to ensure these continue to be embedded in healthcare delivery.

Family medicine's role in society and health systems

The World Health Organisation (WHO) views primary healthcare as the cornerstone of sustainable healthcare systems and emphasises that FM is the key provider. The 1978 WHO Alma Ata Declaration, reaffirmed by the Astana Declaration of 2018, commits the global community to the leading principle of "Health for All", to ensure social justice, equity, and solidarity in healthcare. This should be achieved primarily through strong primary care.[14]

The well-trained family doctor has become a key figure, and often a leader, in the organisation of healthcare. Horizontal and vertical integration of the undergraduate curriculum can be achieved through FM. Horizontally, integration is achieved by family doctors working as team members with other health professionals and in collaboration with community support services. Vertical integration is achieved by collaboration across the three levels of care, as patients move through the healthcare system.

The shaping of FM as an academic discipline began in the1960s and is described in Chapter 5. This has helped focus attention directly on the relationship between these viable FM working principles and values, enabling recognition of this branch of medical practice as a specialty. Medical students should understand its place in healthcare delivery and policy and within the organisation of clinical training.

> Medical students should understand the important role of primary healthcare within sustainable healthcare systems to achieve UHC.

Conclusion

FM principles and core values should guide the development of, and be integrated into, the undergraduate curriculum to benchmark standards for primary healthcare. As a FM educator, it is crucial to promote, with passion, FM as a career choice for medical students as well as residents and colleagues. Exposure to, and spending time in, family practice settings is required to ensure all students graduate with an understanding of the principles and values underpinning FM.

References

1. Loudon IS. James Mackenzie Lecture: The origin of the general practitioner. J R Coll Gen Pract. 1983;33(246):13–23.
2. Vicente VC. History of family medicine over the past 50 years: Global and European perspectives. Available from: https://amf-semfyc.com/web/article/2232 (Accessed 22 August 2022).
3. Jamoulle M, Resnick M, Stichele van der R, Ittoo A, Cardillo E, Vanmeerbeek M. Analysis of definitions of general practice, family medicine, and primary health care: A terminological analysis. BJGP Open. 2017;1(3). doi: 10.3399/bjgpopen17X101049
4. McWhinney I. Principles of family medicine. In: Ian McWhinney R. (ed.), A textbook of family medicine. 2nd ed. Oxford: Oxford University Press; 1997. p. 13.
5. The role of the general practitioner/family physician in health care systems: A statement from WONCA. 1991. Available from: https://medfamcom.files.wordpress.com/2009/10/wonca-statement-1991.pdf (Accessed 22 August 2022)
6. Kelly L. Four principles of family medicine. Do they serve us well? Can Fam Physician. 1997;43:1902–04.
7. Michels NR, Maagaard R, Svab I, Scherpbier N. Teaching and learning core values in General Practice/Family Medicine: A narrative review. Front Med (Lausanne). 2021; 8: 647223. doi: 10.3389/fmed.2021.647223.
8. Sigurdsson JA, Beich A, Stavdal A. A saga-in-progress: Challenges and milestones on our way toward the Nordic core values and principles of family medicine/general practice. Front Med.2021;8:681612. doi: 10.3389/fmed.2021.681612
9. Lawson HJO, Nortey DNN. Core values of family physicians and general practitioners in the African context. Front Med. 2021;8:667144. doi:10.3389/fmed.2021.667144
10. Europe WONCA. The European definition of general practice/family medicine. https://www.woncaeurope.org/file/520e8ed3-30b4-4a74-bc35-87286d3de5c7/Definition3rd%20ed%202011%20with%20revised%20wonca%20tree.pdf. (Accessed 22 August 2022).
11. Pereira-Gray DJ, Sidaway-Lee K, White E, Thirne A, Evans P. Continuity of care with doctors: A matter of life and death? A systematic review of continuity of care and mortality. BMJ Open. 2017. http://dx.doi.org/10.1136/bmjopen-2017-021161
12. McCracken EC, Stewart MA, Brown JB, McWhinney IR. Patient-centred care: The family practice model. Can Fam Physician. 1983;29:2313–16.
13. McWhinney IR. Teaching the principles of family medicine. Can Fam Physician. 1981;27:801–04.
14. Rawaf S, De Maeseneer J, Starfield B. From Alma-Ata to Almaty: A new start for primary health care. Lancet. 2008;372(9647):1365–67.

3

Social accountability

Maham Stanyon, Leilanie Nicodemus, and Robin Ramsay

SUMMARY OF KEY LEARNING POINTS

- Social accountability (SA) unites education, health service provision, and workforce distribution in partnership with communities to meet population health needs and address health inequity.
- SA in education requires the measurement of curriculum outputs with review and action focused on community impact, a key part of quality improvement.
- SA must be defined locally to integrate socially accountable practice within existing family medicine (FM) education systems.
- It is important to recognise, celebrate, and incentivise socially accountable practice locally to support a strong SA culture.
- Open-access sharing of good practice and international academic mentorship can build global networks to foster socially accountable curriculum transformation worldwide.

The need for social accountability in health professions education

The 21st century global healthcare challenges have accelerated the need to reform the traditional biomedical medical school curriculum.[1] SA is now identified as central to training a viable healthcare workforce for the future and achieving universal health coverage (UHC).[2] At all levels of training, SA must be compatible with competency and value-based educational models if UHC milestones are to be realised. If this is achieved, it provides a framework for education and healthcare reform which is adaptable to low-, middle-, and high-income countries.[3]

> A socially accountable curriculum is key to training a viable healthcare workforce and for achieving universal health coverage.

DOI: 10.1201/9781003325734-4

What is social accountability?

Emerging in 1995 from the four pillars of healthcare delivery[4]—equity, quality, efficiency and relevance—SA has evolved into a measurable process which improves population healthcare outcomes by uniting education delivery and health service provision to address health inequity challenges in the communities served.[5] SA can be represented as a gradient of social obligation[3] when addressing community needs. This marks the transition of obligation from "awareness of" (social responsibility) and "action on" (social responsiveness) to an explicitly socially accountable process of healthcare outcome measurement (see Box 3.1). The new SA mandate can drive a sustainable cycle of quality improvement.[2]

Translated into medical education, indicators can be developed to measure how curriculum outputs address community health priorities setting actions to maximise community impact. This must be supported by institutional systemic change and community partnership. The curriculum process embraces multiple aspects of health education delivery, ranging from student selection through to graduation outcomes. All have the power to contribute to and reduce health inequity, depending on how they are used and viewed within. Outcomes need to be socially accountable to every aspect of curricular influence, from clinical services and workforce to research priorities. SA should be viewed as a continuous quality improvement process across the curriculum. It must contextualise high-quality learning, teaching, and equitable service delivery to articulate and implement the professional values of modern healthcare.

> Social accountability implements the professional values of modern healthcare in a continuous quality improvement process for high-quality learning, teaching, and equitable service delivery.

BOX 3.1   KEY DEFINITIONS FOR UNDERSTANDING SOCIAL ACCOUNTABILITY

Term	Definition
Equity	The allocation of support (e.g. resources, workforce, research) depending on need within a population to achieve access to quality healthcare
Social responsibility	Cognisance of the obligation to respond to the needs within a population
Social responsiveness	Taking action to address the needs within a population
Social accountability	A systematic process of engagement with communities to ensure that education and healthcare delivery positively impact health system performance and population health status with measured outcomes feeding into a sustainable cycle of quality improvement

(Adapted from Boelen et al and Clithero et al.[2,3])

Transferring socially accountable principles globally across healthcare systems

New or revised curricula should incorporate SA as an important vertical theme across all years. Yet, despite providing a foundation for curricular reform grounded in universal principles and global health development goals, SA is struggling to cross cultures and impact on educational reform.[6,7] The following are the common challenges encountered when incorporating SA into curricular design:

1. *Terminology:* English is commonly used to exchange educational ideas. It is unfortunately not always possible to accurately translate concepts and words into other languages. This leads to difficulty in understanding the terminology around SA. For example, there are cultures where *responsibility* and *accountability* are not linguistically distinguished.[7] Terms may lose intrinsic meaning when translated. The lack of a shared frame of reference limits the efficacy of discussions and hinders the spread of "SA" as a term within local vocabularies. This impacts on the recognition of existing socially accountable practice.

2. *The biomedical approach to healthcare system design and education:* In healthcare systems where patients have free access to specialist secondary and tertiary care facilities, the biomedical disease–based model prevails. Social, community-orientated needs are not necessarily addressed.[7] Furthermore, education systems based on a biomedical disease model risk disconnecting medical schools from their communities. Case 1 (Box 3.2) illustrates how a "step ladder-type" curriculum integrates education with community service delivery.[8,9]

3. *Progress in primary healthcare development:* A healthcare workforce equipped to deliver community-embedded education and clinical care is essential. Countries where primary healthcare is poorly developed may lack this workforce. The community health faculty risks becoming disproportionately underrepresented, reducing opportunities for community teaching and formal links to community-based services. This denies students authentic and contextualised learning of socially accountable practice from visible FM role models. Case 1 (Box 3.2) illustrates how to capacity-build a workforce for remote areas by widening access and return-service agreements.

4. *Lack of congruency with context:* The local context may lack a culture of quality improvement and quality management frameworks. Cultural differences in forming relationships between stakeholders, the impact of power structures, and the political environment can affect the agency of individuals and institutions to initiate change. Lack of alignment with funding, promotion, and reward pathways further disincentivise moves towards SA, compounded by lack of access to global networks and international support.

An inadequate community workforce and lack of congruency with local contexts challenge the implementation of SA.

BOX 3.2 CASE STUDIES FROM A DEVELOPING COUNTRY WHERE A SOCIALLY ACCOUNTABLE CURRICULUM ADDRESSES SPECIFIC POPULATION HEALTH CHALLENGES

Case 1: The School of Health Sciences (SHS) in Palo, Leyte, Philippines

In the Philippines, implementing SA strategies to improve human resource development and address maldistribution of the health workforce is a priority. The SHS was established in 1976 to produce a health workforce to serve the country's depressed and underserved areas. The school developed a primary care/community-based curriculum for all health professions.[8,9]

Two outstanding features relevant to social equity are as follows:

1. *Preferential student selection from lower socio-economic rural and remote communities:* Recruitment, retention, and capacity-building were aligned to community needs. Communities with a dearth of health workers are involved in nominating applicants. Students commit on entry to serve the community after training. National academic admission requirements are waived.[9]

2. *Learning occurs within the healthcare system:*[9] The stepladder-type curriculum for midwives, nurses, and physicians is community-based, integrating community service provision through projects at each education stage.[8,9] Graduates must render healthcare services in their respective communities, with a two-year return-service agreement for each year of scholarship. This model has a proven 95% graduate retention rate in distant rural areas, particularly among midwives and nurses.[9]

Case 2: Ateneo de Zamboanga University School of Medicine, Zamboanga, Philippines

This school founded its education on serving the poorest and most isolated communities in Zamboanga through its Medicine–Public Health (MD-MPH) programme. Their vision was operationalised by targeting faculty development competencies, programme learning outcomes, and curricular content to improve population health outcomes. Analysis using THEnet Evaluation Framework[12] and the WHO's recommended "6 Building Blocks of quality health systems"[18] showed that longitudinal community engagement and community immersion in the final year provided a rich learning environment for students to develop competencies oriented towards addressing social determinants of health.[19]

Priorities for adapting social accountability to your context

1. *Contextualise terminology and examine the local context:* Use terminology and definitions that convey meaning relevant to your local context. This generates awareness and engages institutions, academic networks, and stakeholders. Identify practical examples of SA in your context.

2. *Establish your institution's position:* Use frameworks such as the International Federation of Medical Students' Associations (IFMSA) Students' Toolkit[10]

BOX 3.3 THEnet EVALUATION FRAMEWORK PHASES AND ACCOMPANYING KEY QUESTIONS

What needs are we addressing?	Who do we serve? What are the needs of the communities that we serve? What are the needs of our health system?
How do we work?	What do we believe in? How do we work with others? How do we make decisions? How do we manage resources?
What do we do?	Who are the educators and how are they trained? Who are our learners? What do our learners learn? How do our learners learn? Where do our learners learn? What contribution do we make to the delivery of healthcare? Does our research programme relate to the mission and values of social accountability?
What difference do we make?	Where are our graduates? What are our graduates doing? How do we support our graduates and other health workers? How have we shared our ideas and influenced others? What impact have we made with other schools? What differences have we made to the health of communities and regions that we serve? What difference have we made to the health system in our region?

(From THEnet online[12])

Each star shows how definition, collaboration, and integration aid transfer from theory to practice.

Assess who	• Define the community and key stakeholders for collaboration • Integrate as partners for joint undertaking of all cycle stages
Identify needs	• Define needs of all partners • Collaborate to identify common goals • Integrate into joint objectives
Deliver service learning	• Define how planned outputs will meet needs • Collaborate to ensure feedback from all stakeholders and integrate into service delivery
Evaluate outcomes	• Define outcomes in terms of meeting needs addressed • Collaborate with partners to review feedback • Integrate into a review of overall process
Adjust for sustainability	• Define where needs have/have not been met • Collaborate to refine stages for improved outcomes • Integrate recommendations into next cycle

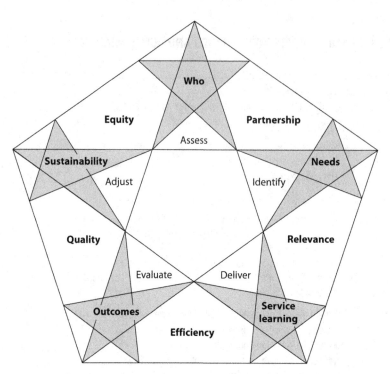

DIAGRAM 3.1 An adapted version of THEnet Member School's Social Accountability Operational Model.[13] The key processes *assess, identify, deliver, evaluate,* and *adjust* are contextualised by five supporting grey stars, to add direction and focus. *Adapted from THEnet online.*[15]

and the Indicators of Social Accountability Tool (ISAT).[11] ISAT offers regular assessment of progress using SA to optimise medical school outputs and identify priority areas. Workforce challenges may limit the uptake of socially accountable practice. This is dependent on healthcare and education design which must view SA as a multi-stakeholder-driven directional change to orient and optimise services to community needs. Thus, it enables all cultures to make progress with existing resources despite differences in UHC achievement.

3. *Use existing education development opportunities for socially accountable reform:* Concurrent curriculum value and competency-based reform enables outcomes to be measured in terms of SA Frameworks such as the Training for Health Equity Network (THEnet) Evaluation Framework[12] and the ISAT tool[11] which can map the entire process, supporting critical performance review, indicator development, and verification of outcomes.

4. *Aim for institutional accreditation recognising SA as a marker of distinction:* The "ASPIRE Recognition of Excellence in SA of a Medical School" offers one such international accreditation framework.[13] Building SA into research grant funding criteria and career promotion pathways further incentivises its progression.

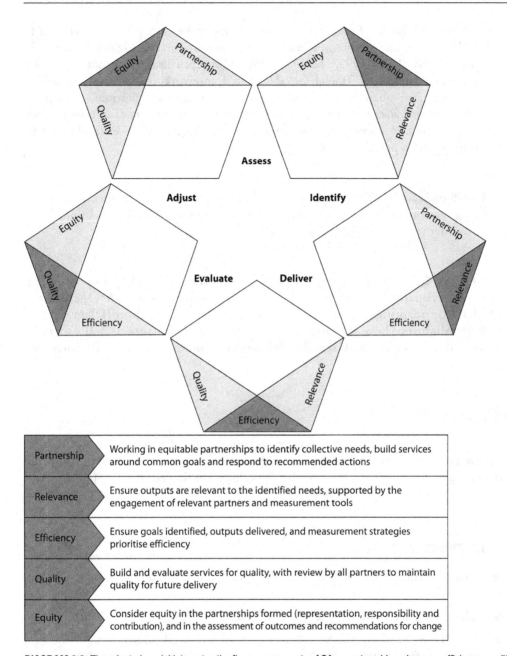

DIAGRAM 3.2 The adapted model integrates the five core concepts of SA—*partnership, relevance, efficiency, quality,* and *equity*—prioritising these at each cycle stage (shown in black) and demonstrating overlap with adjacent concepts (grey). *Adapted from THEnet Online.*[15]

5. *Seek out and share good practice:* Share local examples through open access publishing where possible. Global networks, such as THEnet and The Network Towards Unity for Health (TUFH), can support SA transformation and bring institutions and resources together by sharing vision.

6. *THEnet Evaluation Framework and the Member School's SA Operational Model:* THEnet Evaluation Framework was developed using a logical framework matrix (NORAD 1999)[2] based on the "Conceptualisation, Production and Usability" model of Boelen et al.[14] The framework is a critical, iterative, validated four-phase review process. Each phase asks key questions, guided by *aims* and *indicators* to verify achievement and highlight *sources of evidence* and tools. Box 3.3 shows the framework. Case 2 (Box 3.2) exemplifies the framework in practice.

> Use of tools such as THEnet Evaluation Framework and the Member School's Social Accountability Operational Model can support socially accountable curricular transformation.

THEnet Evaluation Framework[12] uses a continuous quality improvement approach, visually representing the processes involved in an SA Operational Model.[15] By adapting this model to support practical application (Diagram 3.1) and highlighting how to prioritise key principles (Diagram 3.2), socially accountable teaching and service delivery outcomes can be built into the curriculum.

Conclusion

SA can transform curricula to improve community health outcomes and reduce health inequity. Inclusivity, to support global uptake, requires the identification and negotiation of cultural and systemic barriers alongside the sensitive, supported integration of contextualised frameworks.

Key documents

- AMEE Guide 109: Producing a Socially Accountable Medical School (2016)[3]

- The Social Accountability of Medical Schools and Its Indicators (2012)[16]

- Global Consensus for the Social Accountability of Medical Schools (2010)[17] (Available from: https://wfme.org/home/projects/social-accountability/)

Tools

- **IFMSA Video and Social Accountability Toolkit**[10] (Available from: https://ifmsa.org/social-accountability/)

- **ISAT Tool**[11] (Available from: https://socialaccountabilityhealth.org/)

- **THEnet Evaluation Framework**[12]
  (Available from: https://thenetcommunity.org/the-framework/)

- **THEnet Member School's Social Accountability Operational Model/ Continuous Quality Improvement Model**[15]
  (Available from: https://thenetcommunity.org/framework-introduction/)

- **ASPIRE Recognition of Excellence in Social Accountability of a Medical School**[13]
  (Available from: https://amee.org/amee-initiatives/aspire#Social-Accountability-of-the-School)

References

1. Fitzgerald M, Shoemaker E, Ponka D, et al. Global health and social accountability: An essential synergy for the 21st century medical school. J Glob Health. 2021;11:03045.
2. Clithero A, Ross SJ, Middleton L, et al. Improving community health using an outcome-oriented CQI approach to community-engaged health professions education. Front Public Health. 2017;5(26). Available from: https://www.frontiersin.org/articles/10.3389/fpubh.2017.00026/full (Accessed November 2021).
3. Boelen C, Pearson D, Kaufman A, et al. Producing a socially accountable medical school: AMEE guide no. 109. Med Teach. 2016;38(11):1078–91. doi: 10.1080/0142159X.2016.1219029.
4. Boelen C, Heck JE. Defining and measuring the social accountability of medical schools. World Health Organisation [Internet]. 1995. Available from: https://apps.who.int/iris/handle/10665/59441 (Accessed October 2021).
5. Prihatiningsih TS, Kamal Y, Woollard R, et al. Social accountability and accreditation: Impacting health system performance and population health. Soc Innov J. 2020;3. Available from: https://socialinnovationsjournal.com/index.php/sij/article/view/528 (Accessed December 2021).
6. Preston R, Larkins S, Taylor J, et al. Building blocks for social accountability: A conceptual framework to guide medical schools. BMC Med Educ. 2016;16:227. Available from: https://doi.org/10.1186/s12909-016-0741-y (Accessed November 2021).
7. Ramsay R, Stanyon M, Takahashi N. Social accountability across cultures, does the concept translate? An explorative discussion with primary care colleagues in Japan. Educ Prim Care. 2020;31(2):66–70. doi: 10.1080/14739879.2020.1727780
8. Siega-Sur JL, Woolley T, Ross SJ, et al. The impact of socially accountable, community-engaged medical education on graduates in the Central Philippines: Implications for the global rural medical workforce. Med Teach. 2017;39(10):1084–91.
9. Sana EA, Atienza MA, Salvacion MLDS, et al. Transformative scale-up of the school of health sciences, university of the Philippines Manila. Philippine J Health Res Dev. 2019;23(1):16–28.
10. International Federation of Medical Students' Association (IFMSA). Students' Toolkit on Social Accountability in Medical Schools [Internet]. Available from: https://ifmsa.org/social-accountability/ (Accessed December 2021).
11. Social Accountability Health Website. The Institutional Self-Assessment Social Accountability Tool (ISAT) [Internet]. Available from: https://socialaccountabilityhealth.org/ (Accessed December 2021).
12. THEnet Website. THEnet Evaluation Framework [Internet]. Available from: https://thenetcommunity.org/the-framework/ (Accessed December 2021).

13. ASPIRE International Recognition of Excellence in Education Website. ASPIRE Recognition of Excellence in Social Accountability of a Medical School [Internet]. Available from: https://www.aspire-to-excellence.org/Areas±of±Excellence/ (Accessed December 2021).

14. Boelen C, Woollard R. Social accountability and accreditation: A new frontier for educational institutions. Med Educ. 2009;43:887–94.

15. THEnet Website. THEnet Member School's Social Accountability Operational Model/Continuous Quality Improvement Model [Internet]. Available from: https://thenetcommunity.org/framework-introduction/ (Accessed December 2021).

16. Boelen C, Dharamsi S, Gibbs T. The social accountability of medical schools and its indicators. Educ Health. 2012;25:180–94. Available from: https://www.educationforhealth.net/text.asp?2012/25/3/180/109785 (Accessed October 2021).

17. Health Social Accountability Website. Global Consensus for Social Accountability of Medical Schools [Internet]. Available from: http://www.healthsocialaccountability.org (Accessed November 2021).

18. World Health Organisation Website. Monitoring the Building Blocks of Health Systems: A Handbook of Indicators and Their Measurement Strategies [Internet]. Available from: https://apps.who.int/iris/bitstream/handle/10665/258734/9789241564052-eng.pdf (Accessed November 2021).

19. Guignona M, Halili S, Cristobal F, et al. A curriculum for achieving universal health care: A case study of Ateneo de Zamboanga University School of Medicine. Front Public Health. 2021;9:439. https://www.frontiersin.org/articles/10.3389/fpubh.2021.612035/full

4

Developing an appropriate workforce for the future

Archna Gupta and Raman Kumar

SUMMARY OF KEY LEARNING POINTS

- Under-investment in the education and training of health workers, particularly in primary care, contributes to the ongoing workforce shortages.
- Family medicine (FM) must be included as a core component of the undergraduate medical curriculum to ensure exposure to the field for all physicians.
- Evidence shows that greater exposure to FM during the undergraduate medical curriculum leads to more students choosing a career in the specialty.
- To ensure a sustainable workforce for the generations to come, nations, governments, and medical education institutions should prioritise the education and training of family physicians which must begin at the undergraduate level.

Healthcare workforce

The health workforce is a vital contributor to the performance and sustainability of health systems. Improving health service coverage to achieve high care standards and, ultimately, Universal Health Care (UHC), depends on the availability, accessibility, acceptability, and quality of the workforce.[1] Simply having more health workers is not sufficient. Health workers need to be equitably distributed and accessible to the population. They must have the required competency, be motivated, and empowered to deliver quality care which is acceptable to the sociocultural expectations of the people and supported by the health system.[1]

The World Health Organisation projects a shortfall of 18 million health workers by 2030, primarily in low- and middle-income countries (LMICs).[1] However, countries of all socio-economic development face difficulties in education, employment, retention, and workforce performance.[1] Under-investment in the education and training of health workers contributes to the ongoing shortages.[1]

DOI: 10.1201/9781003325734-5

The primary healthcare system and its workforce

When considering the effectiveness of a nation's healthcare system, it is essential to look at its primary healthcare (PHC) system. PHC maximises the level and distribution of health and well-being by simultaneously addressing three elements: (i) primary care and essential public health functions as the core of integrated health services; (ii) multisectoral policy and action; and (iii) empowering people and communities.[2]

The PHC workforce includes all occupations engaged in providing health promotion, disease prevention, treatment, rehabilitation and palliative care services, the public health workforce, and those involved in addressing the social determinants of health.[2]

PHC is the most equitable, effective, and cost-effective way to enhance the health of populations.[2] Studies show that PHC reduces the leading causes of morbidity and mortality globally, including maternal, neonatal, and child mortality and deaths from causes such as HIV/AIDS, malaria, tuberculosis, and vaccine-preventable diseases.[3] It reduces total healthcare costs, increases efficiency by improving access to preventative and promotive services, provides earlier diagnosis and treatment for many conditions, delivers care that focuses on the whole person's needs, and reduces avoidable hospital admissions.[4,5]

Many of the core interventions benefiting PHC relate to primary care.[3,6]

> The PHC workforce includes all professions engaged in health at a population level while primary care is driven by healthcare providers who deliver first contact, continuous, comprehensive, and coordinated care to populations.

Primary care and its workforce

Primary care is "first-contact, continuous, comprehensive, and coordinated care provided to populations undifferentiated by gender, disease, or organ system".[4] The four main features of primary care services are (i) first-contact access for each new need; (ii) long-term person (not disease)-focused care; (iii) comprehensive care for most health needs; and (iv) coordinated care when it is sought elsewhere. Based on the landmark research by Starfield, the global community judges primary care as "good" according to how well these four features are fulfilled.[4]

Family physicians, general practitioners (GPs), and non-physician primary care providers deliver primary care services. Non-physician primary care providers are a broad group, including, but not limited to, lay or community health workers, nurses, physician assistants, midwives, social workers, and pharmacists.

The evidence that primary care contributes to better health in high-income countries is strong. Populations with access to "good" primary care have better health outcomes.[4] Evidence shows that higher numbers of family or primary care doctors are associated with earlier disease detection and decreased mortality rates and premature deaths. These include various preventable conditions, e.g. asthma, cardiac, and cerebrovascular diseases.[7] In LMICs, populations with primary care programmes have better access to healthcare, decreased health costs, and improved health outcomes, including minimising wealth-based disparities in mortality.[3,8]

Family medicine and its relationship to primary care and primary healthcare

Primary care is further strengthened by FM physicians. FM is a subset of primary care as shown in Figure 4.1.[9] Given the diversity and breadth of family physicians' roles, they often straddle the primary and secondary care sectors, depending on their work context.

FM follows eight core principles that guide its education and training—access or first-contact care, comprehensiveness, continuity of care, coordination, prevention, family orientation, community orientation, and patient-centeredness. Noteworthy, four of the eight principles overlap with the components of good primary care.[9]

The delivery, organisation, and management of health services by family physicians distinguish FM from primary care.

Globally, healthcare systems continue to struggle as gaps in delivery and inequities in access widen.[10] At the same time, we face increasing infectious and

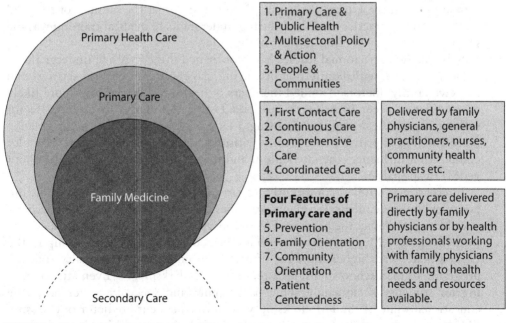

FIGURE 4.1 Relationship between family medicine, primary care, and primary healthcare.[9]

environmental health risks and demographic and epidemiological shifts further stressing the healthcare system and workforce.[10] The medical professional education system has not kept pace with the current challenges, primarily due to fragmented and outdated curricula that produce graduates ill-equipped to manage the complex patient and population needs.[10]

> One way of addressing increasingly complex health problems is by strengthening the primary care workforce, particularly, training family doctors.

Supporting undergraduate family medicine training

To understand FM and generalism (Chapter 1), it is essential that FM is included as a core component of the undergraduate medical curriculum. This supports having a cadre of undergraduate medical students interested in a career in the field and working in primary care. It encourages a strong appreciation for the role of FM and primary care in the health system, by both those who choose to enter FM and those who choose to specialise in other disciplines.

The importance of exposure to family medicine in medical schools

Considerable evidence highlights the link between exposure to FM in the undergraduate curriculum and students choosing a career in the field. A review study from 1995 looking at factors that promote medical students choosing a career in primary care in the United States and Canada found that the number of required weeks of family practice clerkships during undergraduate medical training was the strongest factor for choosing a career in the field.[11]

Subsequent international studies have confirmed this.[12,13] When undergraduate students interact with family doctors in the classroom and clinical settings and perceive family doctors as valued members of health teams, they are more likely to consider a career in primary care and FM.[14,15] Similarly, an essential factor influencing medical students choosing a career in primary care is the relative representation of primary care faculty within an educational institution.[11] Faculty composition influences the curriculum and shapes other faculty's attitudes about generalist specialties.[11]

International studies consistently report that undergraduate FM clerkships positively improve medical students' attitudes towards FM. The clerkship experience helps counteract the negative FM stereotypes of low status and intellectually unchallenging.[16] Medical schools with a required third-year FM clerkship in the United States had higher numbers of graduates entering FM specialty training programmes than schools without a required FM clerkship.[17–19] Even after adjusting for students' sociodemographic background and specialty preferences, the educational value of the FM clerkship was an independent predictor of choosing FM specialty training.[16] Greater exposure to FM, preceptorships, clerkships, or internships in FM and positive FM role models positively influence medical students to enter the field.[12,20]

There is strong international evidence that exposure to FM in the undergraduate curriculum increases the likelihood of students considering a career in FM.

Beyond simply exposure to FM at medical school, it is important that FM is presented and integrated into the curriculum. Traditionally, undergraduate medical education training has occurred through organ-focused disciplines in secondary care hospital settings. Meanwhile, "90% of all patient contacts happen in the community".[20] There is recognition that medical school learning should move away from "fixed rotations through specialties" to more longitudinal attachments where students follow patients through the different areas of healthcare predominantly seen in primary care.[20]

The findings from these studies highlight the importance of having a strong FM presence, including a formal FM curriculum and positive FM experiences alongside family physician teachers and mentors in undergraduate medical programmes.

"Every medical school in the world should have an academic department of family medicine/general practice/primary care. And every medical student in the world should experience family medicine/general practice/primary career as early as possible and as often as possible in their training".

—WONCA Singapore Statement of 2007

Countries where FM is emerging

Many countries globally have been introducing FM over time.[9] In the 1980s, Brazil, Chile, Venezuela, Lebanon, Sri Lanka, Nepal, Thailand, Uganda, and Nigeria initiated FM training followed by Uruguay, Turkey, India, and Vietnam in the 1990s. Since 2000, many Sub-Saharan African countries have implemented FM training, including Ghana, Botswana, Kenya, Nigeria, Lesotho, Ethiopia, Malawi, and Zimbabwe. Typically, postgraduate FM training programmes are first introduced. However, it is now well established that all medical students must be exposed to solid integration of FM in medical school curricula (Chapter 11) with strong, visible support from faculty and across the institution to ensure they consider FM as a career.

India is one such example. Postgraduate FM training was introduced in the early 1980s and significant strides to increase training and production of family physicians have resulted over the last decade. A critical facilitator has been the Academy of Family Physicians of India (AFPI) since it was established in 2010 with the mandate of engaging political leadership, bureaucracy, higher judiciary, and other stakeholders to develop a distinct FM academic discipline. A focus area has been advocacy for the introduction and scale-up of FM in the undergraduate curriculum. Box 4.1 outlines the journey.

> ### BOX 4.1 INTRODUCING FM INTO UNDERGRADUATE (UG) MEDICAL TRAINING IN INDIA
>
> **1983** FM recognised as a postgraduate medical specialty by Medical Council of India but NO mandate for FM in UG medical curricula.
>
> **1983** Medical Education Review Committee, set up by Ministry of Health (MoH) and Family Welfare, Government of India, recommended "medical students be posted in general practice outpatient units and FM developed to increase students pursuing this area".
>
> **2002** National Health Policy outlined a need for expertise in Public Health and FM.
>
> **2003** A WHO SEARO Regional Scientific Working Group Meeting on the FM Core Curriculum convened and recommended the incorporation of FM in UG medical curricula.
>
> **2007** Indian Prime Minister's National Knowledge Commission stated that medical education needs a strong base of basic scientists and clinical generalists/FM specialists.
>
> **2013** A national consultation by the National Rural Health Mission, MoH and Family Welfare, in partnership with AFPI, recommended the central government, state governments, and universities implement the Indian government's FM policy.
>
> **2017** National Health Policy emphasised the need to popularise FM to attract and retain medical doctors in rural areas and create continuing medical education options. This was linked to the Indian government's Health Minister participation in the 2015 AFPI conference.
>
> **2018** AFPI filed public interest litigation with the Supreme Court of India to support implementing FM programmes. Under the direction of the Court, AFPI approached the Government and the Medical Council of India again.[21] AFPI received written assurance from the Prime Minister's office that FM would be included in the 2019 National Medical Commission Act.
>
> **2019** National Medical Commission Act 2019 passed by Indian Parliament mandating UG boards develop dynamic competency-based curricula addressing PHC services, community, and FM. This was not applied to any other discipline.
>
> **2019** A Specialist Board in FM created under National Board of Examinations, MoH, Government of India. National curriculum for FM PG training published in 2021.
>
> **2020** A new one-month foundation course implemented in UG MBBS programmes across the country to include 1 hour dedicated to FM principles.[22]

The AFPI continues to advocate for every medical school to have a distinct, independent FM department under the mandate of the 2019 National Medical Commission. In 2022, the AFPI organised a national consultation, including governments and other stakeholders, to develop a national curriculum similar to that achieved in 2021 for postgraduate training. Resources have subsequently been prepared to support growth of undergraduate FM, including (i) a standardised FM curriculum; (ii) assessment and evaluation metrics; (iii) clinical rotations; (iv) internships; and (v) development of FM departments with minimum standards for infrastructure and faculty. These resources have been submitted to the Ministry of Health and National Medical Commission.

Ensuring a sustainable workforce for the future

As nations work globally towards achieving UHC, we should recognise the critical roles that generalist primary care providers contribute—including family physicians. PHC and primary care play an essential role in ensuring effective and patient-centred care and reducing healthcare inequities. This requires sustainable and high-quality training of family physicians. To achieve a sustainable workforce for future generations, nations, governments, and medical education institutions should not only prioritise postgraduate FM training but must also ensure all students are adequately exposed to FM while at medical school.

References

1. World Health Organization. Global strategy on human resources for health: Workforce 2030. Geneva, Switzerland. 2020.
2. Dussault G, Kawar R, Castro Lopes S, Campbell J. Building the primary health care workforce of the 21st century. Background paper to the Global Conference on Primary Health Care: From Alma-Ata towards Universal Health Coverage and the Sustainable Development Goals. Geneva: World Health Organization. 2018.
3. Kruk ME, Porignon D, Rockers PC, Van Lerberghe W. The contribution of primary care to health and health systems in low- and middle-income countries: A critical review of major primary care initiatives. Soc Sci Med. 2010;70:904–11.
4. Starfield B, Shi L, Macinko J. Contribution of primary care to health systems and health. Milbank Q. 2005;83(3):457–502.
5. Starfield B. Primary care: An increasingly important contributor to effectiveness, equity and efficiency of health services. Gac Sanit. 2012;26(1):20–26.
6. Macinko J, Starfield B, Shi L. The contribution of primary care systems to health outcomes within Organization for Economic Cooperation and Development (OECD) countries, 1970–1998. Health Serv Res. 2003;38(4):831–65.
7. Gibbon W. Medical schools for the health-care needs of the 21st century. Lancet. 2007;369:2211–13.
8. Macinko J, Starfield B, Erinosho T. The impact of primary healthcare on population health in low- and middle-income countries. J Ambul Care Manage. 2009;32(2):150–71.
9. Gupta A, Steele Gray C, Landes M, Sridharan S, Bhattacharyya O. Family medicine: An evolving field around the world. Can Fam Physician. 2021;67(9):647–51.
10. Frenk J, Chen L, Bhutta ZA, Cohen J, Crisp N, Evans T, et al. Health professionals for a new century: Transforming education to strengthen health systems in an interdependent world. Lancet. 2010;376(9756):1923–58.
11. Bland CJ, Meurer LN, Maldonado G. Determinants of primary care specialty choice: A non-statistical meta-analysis of the literature. Acad Med. 1995;70(7):620–41.
12. Amin M, Chande S, Park S, Rosenthal J, Jones M. Do primary care placements influence career choice: What is the evidence? Educ Prim Care. 2018;29(2):64–7. doi: 10.1080/14739879.2018.1427003
13. Shah A, Gasner A, Bracken K, Scott I, Kelly MA, Palombo A. Early generalist placements are associated with family medicine career choice: A systematic review and meta-analysis. Medical Educ. 2021;55(11):1242–52. doi: 10.1111/medu.14578.
14. Campos-Outcalt D, Senf J, Watkins ASB. The effects of medical school curricula, faculty role models, and biomedical research support on choice of generalist physician careers: A review and quality assessment of the literature. Acad Med. 1995;70(7):611–19.
15. Kidd M. The contribution of family medicine to improving health systems: A guidebook from the World Organization of Family Doctors. 2nd ed. London: Radcliffe Publishing; 2013.
16. Turkeshi E, Michels NR, Hendrickx K, Remmen R. Impact of family medicine clerkships in undergraduate medical education: A systematic review. BMJ Open. 2015;5(8):e008265.

17. Campos-Outcalt D, Senf J. A longitudinal, national study of the effect of implementing a required third-year family practice clerkship or a department of family medicine on the selection of family medicine by medical students. Acad Med. 1999;74(9):1016–20.

18. Kassebaum DG, Haynes RA. Relationship between third-year clerkships in family medicine and graduating students' choices of family practice careers. Acad Med. 1992;67(3):217–19.

19. Stine CC, Sheets KJ, Calonge BN. Association between clinical experiences in family practice or in primary care and the percentage of graduates entering family practice residencies. Acad Med. 1992;67(7):475–77.

20. Wass V, Gregory S, Petty-Saphon K. By choice—not by chance: Supporting medical students towards future GP careers. NHS: Health Education England and Medical School Council UK; 2016. https://www.medschools.ac.uk/media/2881/by-choice-not-by-chance.pdf

21. Kumar R. Advocacy to act—family medicine in health policy: A decade-long journey of the Academy of Family Physicians of India. J Family Med Prim Care. 2020;9(4):1805–10.

22. Medical Council of India. Foundation Course for the Undergraduate Medical Education Programme. Dwarka, New Delhi. 2019.

5

Academic primary care

The importance of family medicine leaders and role models

Chris van Weel and Ryuki Kassai

SUMMARY OF KEY LEARNING POINTS

■ Collecting empirical data on family medicine (FM) practice is essential to demonstrate to others its crucial contribution to healthcare.

■ Academic FM ensures primary care (PC) is understood at societal, institutional, and individual patient care levels.

■ All medical schools should aim to have an academic department of FM and academic leaders as role models for medical students.

■ PC research networks provide evidence to improve community healthcare.

■ Developing academic FM departments is challenging but support from international organisations, e.g. WONCA, can help overcome these.

Why academic family medicine is important

The newly appointed professor of FM at the University of Nijmegen, The Netherlands, had just left his office for his first medical student teaching session, but not yet reached the lecture hall, when the Dean of the medical school received a complaint from the Professor of Paediatrics on the subject of the lecture—rubella—a common childhood disease. Children, as everyone ought to know, were his department and not Family Medicines! Rubella in Dutch is called "red dog"—consequently, the incident, which happened long ago, was always referred to as the incident of the "red dog".

Behind the paediatrician's dismay and academic infighting was a fundamental lack of understanding of FM. In response, the FM department in Nijmegen started to collect, in a systematic way, empirical data and experiences from daily

DOI: 10.1201/9781003325734-6

practice.[1] This clarified the role of FM in rubella and provided evidence of its important role in healthcare. FM doctors intuitively knew this, but it had never been articulated before.

> Collecting empirical data on the contribution made by FM to healthcare is crucial. Academia adds indispensable value to this.

"Red dogs" have haunted PC the world over and have stimulated many places to establish structures to collect empirical data.[2] This has had a substantial impact on the emancipation of FM and PC and on the ability to bridge national borders. Yet, just providing evidence of daily practice was, and will be, insufficient to expel "red dogs" and secure a realistic contribution of FM and PC in health systems. Academic PC and FM leadership is crucial.

Academia adds value to empirical information. This must be seen in the training of future family doctors to enhance evidence-based professional performance, or in research that provides evidence-based guidance compatible with the PC context. Arguably, the most important role of academic teaching is in the early, pre-specialisation phase of medical education. This enables medical students to either make an evidence-based career choice for FM or provide those who will ultimately practise in the hospital setting an understanding of the potential of FM and the importance of collaboration at this interface throughout their career.

> Medical students must understand the importance of academic FM to make evidence-based career choices.

Academic leadership is critical to guide the use of empirical information and experiences to shape the core principles and values of FM in medical schools. This is where the "red dog" operated: It demonstrated ignorance of the value of FM for individual and population health and was driven by assumptions. The paediatric professor assumed that FM doctors operated within the strict limits of his specialist biomedical disease model – and could only perform as the poor cousin of the *real* physician-specialist.

Academic leadership enables medical students to relate data and experiences from everyday FM practice with the overarching values of PC through an integrated bio-psycho-socio-economic approach to the health, illness, and disease of individuals and populations. They need to understand the performance of all PC multi-professional team members and its contribution to society.

At a macro-level, it enables policymakers to understand how PC contributes to the health, stability, and resilience of communities and populations and strengthens the autonomy and self-efficacy of community/patient groups. At the institutional (meso) level, students need to understand how to integrate and place equal value on the competencies of generalism as enacted by FM doctors and hospital-based physicians and specialists.[3] Academic leadership plays an all-important role in broadening a student's understanding of FM above the micro-level, i.e. the application of research to individual patient care. The research underpinning PC must be visible to students.[4]

Academic FM leadership can demonstrate the influence of PC at societal, institutional, and individual patient levels.

We use three examples to illustrate the importance of PC research:

1. *Systematic collection of empirical data from FM practice:* This has shown that, at a population level, people experience health problems with high frequency but only occasionally seek professional healthcare. When professionals do become involved, most problems are dealt with in community PC. Only a small proportion reach specialist hospital care.[5,6] PC deals with 90–95% of all professionally managed health problems, including important chronic conditions, e.g. asthma, chronic obstructive pulmonary disease (COPD), diabetes, and cardiovascular risk management. Yet, traditionally, these chronic conditions are taught by hospital specialists based on the severely affected patients they see, i.e. as little as 5% of all patients—the tip of the iceberg. Students get a skewed perspective of how these conditions commonly present and are managed. Figure 5.1 summarises this "ecology of medical care"

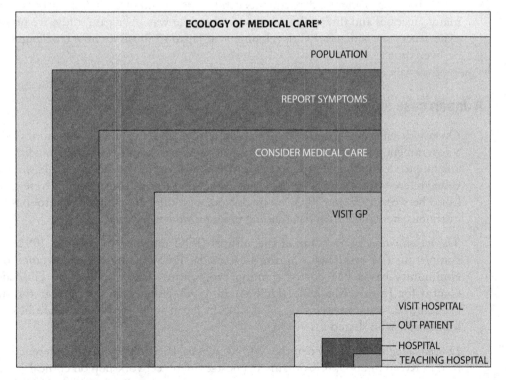

FIGURE 5.1 Ecology of medical care.

illustrating the unique domain of PC-managed health problems vis-à-vis the hospital sector and how social determinants of health impact on defined populations.[7] Although PC professionals recognise this, in our experience, specialist and policymakers often struggle to understand and value it.

2. *Comorbidity:* More than 30 years ago, PC data showed comorbidity or multimorbidity, i.e. individuals often have more than one health problem.[8] FM doctors adopted a person-centred approach to address this in everyday practice. Disease-oriented specialism has taken longer to reconcile with the complexity of multimorbidity.

3. *The paradox of PC:* The contribution of PC to people's health is achieved through more than state-of-the-art treatment of diseases.[9] This—the *paradox of PC*—may agree with the intuitive experiences of FM practitioners but contradicts the basic biomedical disease orientation underpinning medical education. Hence the persistent need for an academic approach to explain FM, and why academic PC has become so important. To understand the strength of evidence supporting PC, departments of FM and academic leaders are needed in every medical school.

Exposure to academic FM is essential to fully understand the reality of PC. Every medical school should have a department of family medicine.

Establishing academic departments can be a long and often tedious process with many successes and disappointments scored on the way. As a case study, we present experiences in academic PC development in Japan to illustrate how challenges can be overcome.

A Japan case study

Overcoming resistance: In 1987, fierce opposition from Japanese medical associations led to a government policy failure to introduce FM doctors to Japan. Poor understanding and a failure to defuse the perception that FM was a threat to the medical establishment's vested interests were contributing factors. Although three PC organisations were established between 1978 and 1993, led by doctors with different clinical backgrounds and intentions, no standardised FM training programme was initiated.

The importance of vision: One of the authors (RK) returned to Japan in 1992 after completing FM residency training in Canada. Recognising the importance of a community-based FM doctor training programme, RK founded the Hokkaido Centre for Family Medicine (HCFM) in 1996, pioneering a four-year training programme. This was the first of its kind in Japan supported by a private hospital foundation who shared his vision.

Disseminating the vision: When the WONCA Asia-Pacific Regional Conference was held in Kyoto in 2005, RK organised a post-conference workshop on clinical education. From this opportunity, momentum for a nationally standardised training programme increased. In 2006, the Japanese Academy of Family Medicine (JAFM) launched a training programme, based on the HCFM model. The JAFM merged with two other PC organisations in 2010, forming the Japan Primary Care Association (JPCA), currently a WONCA member organisation. The training programme evolved accordingly and was accredited in 2019 after achieving the WONCA Global Training Standards for Postgraduate FM Education.[10]

Bringing academic FM into medical schools: Reform at undergraduate level has been slower. Although more than 20 of the 80 Japanese medical schools have established departments of adult "general medicine" since 1981, these have been in tertiary care hospitals disconnected from the community setting. Furthermore, vague terms and definitions of "general medicine" have confused Japanese people, limiting understanding of PC.

> Vague terms and definitions of "generalism" have confused people, limiting understanding of academic family medicine.

After establishing the HCFM as a successful model for postgraduate training, RK moved to Fukushima Medical University in 2006, where he founded the first academic department of PC in Japan. Its initial goals were as follows:

1. Create opportunities for medical students to learn the value of PC.

2. Foster a group of motivated trainers to provide high-quality community-based FM training.

3. Showcase PC as an independent academic discipline that promotes socially accountable research.

The department worked to realise university and government aims, by fostering doctors to serve remote and rural communities. Box 5.1 summarises the added value the department established over 15 years.

PC research networks: One goal was to establish practice-based research networks (PBRNs), an interface between the academic PC/FM department and community teams, to facilitate socially accountable research that prioritises community concerns and translates research outcomes into practice.[11] Practice-based research networks bridge the gap between where care is delivered and where research is conducted, to prioritise important issues, such as health inequity, social determinants of health, and population needs, and to align service delivery accordingly.

In a country like Japan, where the value of PBRNs has not yet been recognised, the support of a dedicated academic PC/FM department is much needed to (i) provide opportunities for community-based healthcare professionals to develop research skills; (ii) revise criteria and support evaluation of research for institutional reviews and research funding bodies; and (iii) support negotiations with policymakers and workforce upskilling. Encouragement in these endeavours from academic family doctors internationally and organisations such as WONCA makes overcoming such challenges less overwhelming.

BOX 5.1 THE ADDED VALUE AN ACADEMIC FAMILY MEDICINE DEPARTMENT BRINGS TO AN INSTITUTION

Categories	Added value
Undergraduate education	Access to the curriculum; student clinical training; involvement in examinations and entry to medical school selection; new curricula with a paradigm shift in healthcare; evidence-based medicine; principles of patient-centred clinical method; training in communication skills and outpatient consultations; FM role models for students; connecting the curriculum with the community
Research support	Access to ethics committees; support with national funding applications for grants; access to library and academic information centres; graduate school education for Masters/PhD students; links with international academic advisors; links with WONCA Working Party on Research; reference for candidates applying for Masters and PhD courses overseas
Vocational training	Operational management of formal FM training programmes (rural and urban communities); train-the-trainers programmes; international study tours; links with WONCA Working Party for Mental Health and International Association for Communication in Healthcare
Organisational/Institutional	International collaboration; hub for exchange programmes and providing international training/working opportunities; Vice Chair of the Conference and Chair of the Scientific Programme Committee of WONCA Asia-Pacific Region Conference 2019; international accreditation of postgraduate training standards

---

Another development goal is capacity-building. Box 5.2 summarises what RK needed to build the department from scratch. Ideally, formal education courses are needed, but we also learnt informally from mistakes. Support from the international community again plays an important role.

> Support from the international community plays an important role in sharing experiences, setting goals, supporting difficult negotiations, and establishing benchmarks.

Finally, PC has been recognised as an essential discipline in Japanese medicine. The Japanese Medical Speciality Board now recognises FM as a specialty and the Japan Accreditation Council for Medical Education has made FM mandatory in undergraduate medical curricula. The COVID-19 pandemic has raised society's expectations for well-trained family doctors in the community.[12]

Hope is always visible. After enduring a long incubation period, academic FM doctors in Japan are taking their place in the reform of Japanese healthcare.

BOX 5.2 WHAT WAS NEEDED TO FOUND THE ACADEMIC PRIMARY CARE DEPARTMENT

Person factors	Vision	Japanese healthcare reforms cannot be accomplished without well-trained family doctors
	Role models	Advice from their experience can support you when under pressure in your context
	Experience	You need experience as a trainee and trainer in PC/FM as a minimum
	Leadership	Knowing how your people want to be led by you
	Resilience	You may have to try many times in vain
	International mentors/advisors	Gracious, thoughtful, and caring teachers to give you support, advice, and encouragement
	International friends/colleagues	Joy can be doubled, and sadness can be shared
Team factors	Initial cohort (trainees, faculty members)	Motivated and committed colleagues can alleviate some of the hardships when starting out
	Multidisciplinary health professionals	Work is more fun when values are shared across disciplines
Institution factors	Needs identification (intrinsic, extrinsic)	Asking "What can the new academic department do for the university and for external partners?"
	Funds	Secure funds are needed to hire initial faculty and trainees
	Teaching practices	Negotiations are needed to satisfy the needs of both parties
Context factors	Momentum	To encourage the public to seek well-trained family doctors and uptake by policymakers

Conclusion

Although the values and contributions of academic FM to the health of individuals and populations may be crystal clear for professionals working in the field, we remain aware that for important parties outside the field, such as hospital specialists and policymakers, this is not the case. Indeed, PC remains an enigma to many. Academic FM must provide the leadership to address this. By openly articulating within medical schools the facts and findings from PC research and providing academic FM leaders to role model PC as a discipline, this can both support hospital specialists, policymakers, and other third parties to understand FM and inspire medical students to become FM doctors.

References

1. Weel CV. The Continuous Morbidity Registration Nijmegen: Background and history of a Dutch general practice database. Eur J Gen Pract. 2008;14(Suppl. 1):5–12.
2. Dania A, Nagykaldi Z, Haaranen A, Muris JWM, Evans PH, Mäntyselkä P, Weel CV. A review of 50 years of international literature on the internal environment of building practice-based research networks (PBRNs). J Am Board Fam Med. 2021;34:762–97. doi: 10.3122/jabfm.2021.04.200595
3. Misky AT, Shah RJ, Yeen Fung C, Sam AH, Meeran K, Kingsbury M, Salem V. Understanding concepts of generalism and specialism amongst medical students at a research-intensive London medical school. BMC Med Educ. 2022;22:291. doi: 10.1186/s12909-022-03355-1
4. Periera Gray D. Towards research-based learning outcomes for general practice in medical schools: Inaugural Barbara Starfield memorial lecture. BJGP Open. 2017;1(1). doi: https://bjgpopen.org/content/1/1/bjgpopen17X100569
5. van de Lisdonk EH. Perceived and presented morbidity in general practice. Scand J Prim Health Care. 1989;7:73–8.
6. Green LA, Fryer GE, Yawn BP, Lanier D, Dovey SM. The ecology of medical care revisited. N Engl J Med. 2001;334:20921–25.
7. Schellevis FG, van der Velden J, van de Lisdonk EH, van Eijk JT, van Weel C. Comorbidity of chronic diseases in general practice. J Clin Epidemiol. 1993;46:469–73.
8. Commission on Social Determinants of Health. Closing the gap in a generation: Health equity through action on the social determinants of health. Geneva, Switzerland: World Health Organization; 2008. http://apps.who.int/iris/bitstream/handle/10665/43943/9789241563703_eng.pdf;jsessionid=4B2D91D4D9AC4E0188108B8C846F953A?sequence=1 (Accessed 23 November 2021).
9. Stange KC, Ferrer RL. The paradox of primary care. Ann Fam Med. 2009;7:293–99.
10. WONCA Postgraduate Training Standards. 2013. Available from: http://www.globalfamilydoctor.com/site/DefaultSite/filesystem/documents/Groups/Education/WONCA%20ME%20stds_edit%20for%20web_250714.pdf
11. Pirotta M, Temple-Smith M. Practice-based research networks. Aust Fam Physician. 2017;46:793–95.
12. Noknoy S, Kassai R, Sharma N, Nicodemus L, Canhota C, Goodyear-Smith F. Integrating public health and primary care: The response of six Asia-Pacific countries to the COVID-19 pandemic. Br J Gen Pract. 2021;71(708):326–29. doi: 10.3399/bjgp21X716417

6

Barriers for change and how to overcome these

Marietjie van Rooyen, Jannie Hugo, and Anselme Derese

SUMMARY OF KEY LEARNING POINTS

■ Raising the profile of family medicine (FM) requires strong championship and determined strategic planning to overcome barriers step by step.

■ Change management is necessary at all levels—political, community healthcare sites, the university, FM faculty, the curriculum, and the student body.

■ Lack of political understanding and acknowledgement of the value of FM at national and local levels needs to be overcome strategically through determined leadership.

■ Creative development of community sites to introduce students to the reality of healthcare, population needs, and social determinants of health has great potential.

■ Working opportunistically with evidence-based objectives to build trust collaboratively with basic science and secondary care teachers aids curriculum change.

■ Using regular quality improvement processes, ensuring inclusivity of all stakeholders, is important to monitor progress and sustain momentum.

Introduction

In most cases, the implementation of FM into the undergraduate curriculum is initiated and driven by dedicated champions. History has shown that this is best done through small changes supported by careful strategic planning, grown incrementally over time. Case studies from the Philippines (Chapter 3), India (Chapter 4), Japan (Chapter 5), and Pakistan (Chapter 11) provide examples of how this has been achieved globally in countries where considerable barriers to change have been overcome. Being aware of significant challenges, harnessing

DOI: 10.1201/9781003325734-7

facilitating influences to catalyse change, and long-term strategic planning are all essential. Continuous evaluation of the programme and key relationships will enable careful proactive planning.[1–3]

> Strongly championed, proactive strategic planning, good communication, and continuous evaluation of the programme and relationships are key factors for successful change.

We have identified five main areas of potential barriers to change that need to be addressed:

- The ministry and governing bodies
- The health system (context of care)
- The university and faculty
- The medical school curriculum
- The FM faculty and the students

Influencing ministry and governing bodies on the importance of family medicine

Recognition of the importance of FM on a national governmental level will significantly assist its establishment as a separate specialty. Globally, especially in some low- and middle-income countries (LMICs), this remains a significant barrier to change. Despite the 2018 Astana Declaration[4] and World Health Organisation (WHO) recognition that primary care is the essential driving force for the successful delivery of Universal Health Care, recognition of the importance of FM by policymakers has been slow.

The incorporation of trained family physicians into the national health system is crucial. Yet, across the world, doctors on graduating from medical school can enter directly into general practice without further training. This is rather ironic given the breadth of knowledge and skill needed to address the increasingly complex challenges of primary health care (Chapter 4). Therefore, working with governments and health policy developers to argue for generalism across all medical education (Chapter 1) and the important role FM can play in delivering this remains, sadly, crucial (Chapter 2).

> Globally, the evidence for the crucial role of primary care still remains unrecognised by some governments and within national healthcare systems. Addressing this is essential.

Box 6.1 summarises these challenges and ways to overcome them.

BOX 6.1 MINISTRY AND GOVERNING BODIES: BARRIERS FOR CHANGE AND FACILITATORS OF CHANGE

Barrier category	Barrier for change	Facilitator of change
Ministry and governing bodies	• Recognition of FM and its role in achieving universal healthcare • Healthcare systems with no postgraduate training for FM • Failure to follow strong evidence supporting the benefits of FM	• Government recognition of FM as a specialty • Incorporation of trained family physicians within national health systems • Development of regional networks • Accreditation of FM training programmes • Inclusion of FM in undergraduate curricula

Determined championing of the evidence for FM as a specialty can drive change. Various strategies do work but are very much dependent on the leadership, local contexts, and national health policies. The development of Academic Departments of FM, mandatory postgraduate training in FM, or inclusion of FM in undergraduate curricula have all proved to be ways to influence governments and policymakers. Regional networks of family physicians will strengthen the process.[5-8]

Working collaboratively with the health system (context of care)

Developing community FM learning opportunities

A significant barrier to change is the perception that undergraduate training should be delivered by hospital specialists. Although specialist training is important, increasingly healthcare is being directed into the community (Chapter 8). A significant part of basic medical education curricula involves preparing students comprehensively to assess patients with undifferentiated presentations and navigate the local healthcare systems. The most appropriate learning platforms for students to achieve these competencies are the health systems' primary care sites. Finding these sites, particularly in LMICs where FM is still developing, can be challenging but very advantageous.

One of the biggest barriers to change is the general perception that undergraduate training needs to happen in hospitals with specialists.

Box 6.2 summarises how change can be achieved.

BOX 6.2 HEALTH SYSTEMS AND CONTEXT OF CARE

Barrier category	Barrier for change	Facilitator of change
Health system (context of care)	• Current health system design and hospital-orientated culture • Establishment of primary care teaching sites • Limited FM services in tertiary hospitals • Balance of service versus learning • Lack of resources, support, and supervision	• Identify FM teaching sites in communities • Stretch care to neglected areas • Develop integrated projects with community care • Align learning between different professionals • Use evaluation to evidence positive investment in the health system • Develop new value-added roles for students • Support and develop the sites to accept students • Solid agreements between university and service delivery sites

Alignment of learning between different professionals

The first initiatives to integrate FM into medical schools arose in countries with healthcare systems where FM had a strong gatekeeping role. In countries where family doctors struggle to gain academic recognition, specialists are equally accessible. Formal relationships between secondary and primary care are lacking. Building understanding at this interface can facilitate collaboration in healthcare and in education.[4,6,7] The interprofessional learning opportunities can also be advantageous when promoting FM; as can sharing resources and space (Chapter 18).

Identify and develop community-based care sites: Students should be exposed to a wide range of healthcare service environments and contexts to develop a holistic understanding of patient and population needs within local health centre systems (Chapter 8). To facilitate FM opportunities, it is important to create real-life learning environments imaginatively. Primary care sites can include FM practices, community-based clinics, old age homes, preschool and day care centres, community hospitals, and community-oriented primary care (COPC) sites.

Stretching care to neglected areas: Although focusing teaching on patients readily available in hospital is easier and less resource intensive, students, often from high socio-economic backgrounds, should be exposed to traditionally neglected groups, e.g. homeless people, informal settlements, lesbian, gay, bisexual, and transgender (LGBTI) communities, substance abuse facilities.

Develop integrated projects with community care: COPC sites bring health professionals and organisations together in defined geographical areas to identify and respond systematically to health needs. Student awareness of the characteristics of community groups vulnerable to disease, potential risk factors, impact of poverty, and thresholds to timely and effective healthcare is often neglected. COPC sites offer opportunities for students to learn from the reality of generalist practice and for FM faculty to collaborate and build community presence.[8] We offer an example:

The University of Pretoria's FM Department (UPFM) saw the national Department of Health's call for the Re-engineering of Primary Health Care in South Africa as an opportunity to enlarge the footprint of FM in the undergraduate curriculum.[9] We built strategically on a local COPC inner city programme addressing the complexity of harmful substance abuse. A community-oriented programme on substance abuse, based on provision of healthcare, education, and research, was introduced for medical students and was well evaluated. By using this existing resource for community projects, we influenced politically and built ongoing collaboration with local services and funders.

Support the sites to accept students: Service delivery is the main objective of any clinical teaching platform and time availability a significant barrier to taking students. It is important that student learning opportunities are structured to benefit both the service and the students. Information, planning, and communication are key factors. Open communication lines for help, information, and building personal relationships add to the success. Community- and home-based healthcare workers or allied healthcare professionals make wonderful facilitators. Longitudinal interprofessional learning relationships between students and workplace teams aid relationships and build trust.[2,6,10,11]

Wide access to community resources enables students to understand population needs and socio-economic reality and strengthens mutual understanding between health professionals.

The role of the university and faculty in facilitating change

There are many ways in which FM faculty can be developed to facilitate change. Box 6.3 summarises these.

Establishing a strong FM faculty: To facilitate change, family doctors must become visible in the undergraduate curriculum acting as respected role models, tutors, and lecturers. The importance of FM academic centres is covered in Chapter 5. Strong leadership is essential to champion change. Faculty programmes for training teachers, on and off campus, can build confidence and education portfolios to support promotion. Central presence on medical school planning sessions is crucial. Positive FM outcomes are more easily achieved if faculty members have strategic roles on all curriculum committees and apply for key appointments such as director of medical education.[4,6]

BOX 6.3 DEVELOPING THE FM FACULTY

Barrier category	Barrier for change	Facilitator of change
Faculty	• Unsupportive faculty leadership • Yearly staff allocation and budget • Lack of expertise • Limited time and effort • Logistical difficulties	• Establishment of FM departments in universities • Leadership explicitly addresses the perception that only physicians can mentor • Provision of training for FM teachers • Faculty development programmes • Career advancement for contribution to teaching • FM faculty members to hold central campus teaching roles in all years • Protected time for teaching • Resources to support and pay teachers • Curriculum implementation team • Centralisation of administrative tasks • Support for research in FM

The medical school curriculum

Box 6.4 summarises ways in which faculty can strategically overcome barriers and gain influence within the curriculum to facilitate change. The following three sections of this book offer much more detailed analysis of the problems and solutions.

The dominance of basic science and hospital specialties is steeped in tradition and can be challenging. Perhaps understandably, the leaders of these curricula perceive any proposition to include others in curriculum structure as a threat, an attack on their "kingdom". Every shift in the curriculum towards more integration of FM content implies "giving in" on territory, lecturing hours, and threatens staff and

BOX 6.4 FACILITATING CHANGE THROUGH THE CURRICULUM

Barrier category	Barrier for change	Facilitator of change
Curriculum	• Traditional curricula with a focus on the basic sciences • Secondary care dominance • Threat of changing roles • Hidden curriculum—the notion that FM is an inferior discipline • Outmoded teaching methods	• Create space in the curriculum • Expose students to FM in all years of training • Important role modelling of generalist expertise • Innovative teaching strategies • Multiple opportunities for interaction with patients • Frequent access to 1:1 supervision with FM tutor • Implementing capability as a learning tool • Opportunities for interprofessional learning • Facilities for longitudinal integrated clerkships

yearly budgets.[4,6] Once again creative, strategic planning gradually building mutual understanding and respect can work. The main challenges are as follows:

Creating space in the curriculum: Fully packed curricula are very common. Strategic design of important FM evidence-based learning outcomes, which are difficult to dispute and best delivered in FM, can aid negotiations.[4,7]

Innovative teaching strategies: The COVID-19 pandemic has impacted significantly on teaching delivery with a strong move to blended learning and opening opportunities for change (Chapter 20). Developing partnerships with specialists instead of taking over their domains, "co-teaching", can work well. Sharing lecturers or case-based discussions, aided by online learning, brings primary and secondary care perspectives together and builds respect and trust. Shared case discussions with all members of the FM can meet curriculum aims for interprofessional learning[6,7] (Chapter 18).

> Suggest partnerships with basic scientists and specialists and avoid any impression of taking over their domains.

Implementing capability as an approach to learning: Capability, as a theoretical framework, works well in the FM environment. It addresses learning in a complex world beyond the acquisition of one competency developing an individual as a professional and a person.[10] Students can be supported to be confident in making judgements and addressing uncertainty and risk in a safe environment (Chapter 24).

Accreditation visits: These can be built on strategically given the global move to more primary care–orientated medical education. An accreditation committee can critique the traditional curriculum, praise new initiatives, and facilitate change.

The FM faculty and the students

Challenges can include students' reluctance to travel and associated expenditure for fares and accommodation. The COVID-19 pandemic widened, especially for LMICs, inequity through lack of access to information technologies and the internet. However, advocating for student inclusiveness by widening access from all backgrounds, especially rural communities, can increase inclusiveness and improve shared peer understanding of disadvantaged backgrounds (Chapter 14). Ensuring learning outcomes are deemed relevant, advantageous, innovative, and carry weight in summative assessments is crucial. If the experience is good, students are generally happy to travel.

Faculty and clinical sites may feel threatened by students reviewing them, but if you use the students as part of the solution it can help. Use the quality improvement cycle (Chapter 31) to make students part of process and involve them in finding creative solutions. Sites generally appreciate feedback. Research is another useful

BOX 6.5 FACILITATING CHANGE THROUGH THE STUDENTS

Barrier category	Barrier for change	Facilitator of change
Student	• Advocating inclusiveness • Unlikely or unwilling to engage because of academic pressure • Lack of baseline skills • Assessment strategies not supportive of learning in primary care sites	• Outreach and admission policies encourage applications from underrepresented communities • Curricula should be sensitive and responsive to the developmental needs of students, by strengthening the teacher–student relationship and providing mentorship as needed • Promote reflective lifelong learning skills with students to identify areas of skill development early • Connect FM system–based experience with learning goals in basic and behavioural sciences

way of addressing challenges and generating funds to support the sites and resources. Focus on evaluating the return of investment to the health system and the impact students have on service delivery.

Regular evaluation, including and supporting all stakeholders, will ensure momentum is sustained and those championing the process remain motivated.

Conclusion

Medical education has been dominated by the traditional hospital-based delivery for a century. It is perhaps not surprising that change to greater community delivery, despite strong evidence it should happen, has been slow. The barriers may be significant, but change is achievable. Strong championship, long-term strategic planning, stakeholder inclusiveness, and creative opportunistic curriculum design can all contribute to change and build collaborative partnerships and mutual inter-professional respect. By monitoring change through regular programme evaluation and celebrating success, however small, progress can be sustained and faculty motivation enhanced.

References

1. Maley M, Worley P, Dent J. Using rural and remote settings in the undergraduate medical curriculum: AMEE guide no 47. Med Teach. 2009;31:969–83.
2. Pipas CF, Peltier DA, Fall JH, Olson AL, Mahoney JF, Skochelak SE et al. Collaborating to integrate curriculum in primary care medical education: Successes and challenges from three US medical schools. Fam Med. 2004;36:S126–S32.

3. Vankatesan S, Prince RHC. Family medicine in undergraduate medical education in India. J Family Med Prim Care. 2014;3(4):300–4.

4. Declaration of Astana and what it means for the global role of NAPCRG and WONCA. Ann Fam Med. 2020;18(2):189–90. doi: 10.1370/afm.2524. PMCID: PMC7062475.

5. Gonzalo JD, Dekhtyar M, Hawkings RE, Wolpaw DR. How can medical students add value? Identifying roles, barriers, and strategies to advance the value of undergraduate medical education to patient care and the health system. Acad Med. 2017;92(9):1294–1301.

6. Family Medicine. Report of a regional scientific working group meeting on core curriculum. Colombo, Sri Lanka. 9–13 July 2003. WHO Project No.: ICP OSD 002 October 2003.

7. Undergraduate Education Committee. Rethinking undergraduate medical education: A view from family medicine. Mississauga, Ontario: The College of Family Physicians of Canada; 2007.

8. Tabatabaei Z, Yazdani S, Sadeghi R. Barriers to integration of behavioral and social sciences in the general medicine curriculum and recommended strategies to overcome them: A systematic review. J Adv Med Educ Prof. 2016;4(3):111–21. https://www.researchgate.net/publication/304701867

9. Marcus TS. A practical guide to doing community oriented primary care. Pretoria, RSA: Department of Family Medicine, University of Pretoria; 2015.

10. Sandars J, Hart CS. The capability approach for medical education: AMEE guide no. 97. Med Teach. 2015;37(6):510–20.

11. Norris TE, Schaad DC, DeWitt D, Ogur B, Hunt DD. Longitudinal integrated clerkships for medical students: An innovation adopted by medical schools in Australia, Canada, South Africa, and the United States. Acad Med. 2009;84(7):902–7.

7

Humanism in family medicine

Martina Kelly and Chandramani Thuraisingham

SUMMARY OF KEY LEARNING POINTS

- Humanist values are based on empathy, reason, and experience and a belief in the welfare of all human beings regardless of race, religion, or nationality.
- Humanism in family medicine (FM) means emphasising the human experience of health and illness.
- Teaching humanism in undergraduate education requires protected curriculum time and institutional commitment.
- Family doctors teach humanism through the following:

  - Role modelling humanism exemplified in caring doctor–patient relationships
  - Collaborative conversations with learners on doctor–patient interactions

- When providing care to a multicultural society, better intercultural understanding, humanistic values, and communication between doctors and patients are needed.

What is humanism?

> *One of the essential qualities of the clinician is interest in humanity, for the secret of the care of the patient is in caring for the patient.*[1]

Humanism is an approach to care that emphasises human values and concerns. Historically, humanism is associated with the Renaissance (1300–1600), when renewed interest in the classical studies from ancient Greece and Rome heralded a move away from religion as the focus of life to emphasise human experience.

DOI: 10.1201/9781003325734-8

Advocates of humanism promoted the study of art, literature, and ancient texts as recognition of human achievements, resulting in the term "humanities", still associated with studying these disciplines.

Humanist values are based on empathy, reason, and experience and a belief in the welfare of all human beings regardless of race, religion, or nationality. In healthcare, humanism is "characterised by a respectful and compassionate relationship between physicians, as well as all other members of the healthcare team, and their patients. It reflects attitudes and behaviours that are sensitive to the values and the cultural and ethnic backgrounds of others".[2] In practice, a wide range of attributes are associated with the ideals of humanism in medical education (Table 7.1), particularly the terms respect, compassion, caring, empathy, and altruism. In addition to being practised by individuals, there is growing recognition of the importance of integrating humanistic values into institutional vision, mission, values, and culture to support system-level humanistic healthcare.[3]

> Humanism is characterised by respectful and compassionate relationships sensitive to the values and cultural and ethnic background of others.

In medical education, humanism is associated with teaching and learning on professionalism, humanities-based activities, and patient-centred care. FM is a clinical discipline which specifically incorporates humanistic approaches to patient care, reflected historically in the work of Enid and Michael Balint, the patient-centred clinical method, and emphasis on bio-psycho-social approaches to patient care.[4] Encouraging and supporting family physicians to discuss and reflect on doctor–patient relationships in the classroom and clinical setting supports integration of humanistic healthcare into undergraduate medical education.

TABLE 7.1 Key attributes of a humanistic healthcare professional ("I.E. C.A.R.E.S.")[2]

Integrity	Congruence between expressed values and behaviour
Excellence	Clinical expertise
Collaboration and compassion	Awareness and acknowledgement of the suffering of another and the desire to relieve it
Altruism	Capacity to put the needs and interests of another before your own
Respect and resilience	Regard for the autonomy and values of another person
Empathy	Ability to put oneself in another's situation, e.g. physician as patient
Service	Sharing one's talent, time, and resources with those in need, giving beyond what is required

Why is humanism important?

Humanistic qualities in physicians help embed trust in the physician–patient relationship, promoting greater adherence to treatment and resulting in improved health outcomes. With use of sophisticated technology in medical practice today, ensuring that a human connection is maintained is more crucial than ever before. Enabling students to learn how to relate to patients early in their training may prevent poor communication and the risk of litigation later in their careers. A humanistic perspective in doctoring instils job satisfaction, intrinsic to physician wellness.[5] For medical students, humanism provides opportunities for self-reflection, raising awareness that patients must be understood in their bio-psycho-sociocultural context.

Why is humanism best acquired in family medicine in the undergraduate curriculum?

The family physician is a "generalist" physician who provides definitive care to the undifferentiated patient at the point of first contact. Family practice, which embeds healthcare processes and the family doctor in meaningful relationships with patients, their families, and communities, within the context of inter-professional teams, is a powerful learning environment for humanism. It is here that students are often confronted by the varying views of less seriously ill patients and their families.

Adopting a bio-psycho-sociocultural approach fosters patient centredness. This is also where students in need of space for personal growth become a part of the social and medical communities where their learning occurs, especially where exemplary "ways of being" are role modelled. Rewards in FM come largely from knowing patients intimately and sharing their trust, respect, and friendship that has developed over time. With each physical or emotional crisis in a patient's life, this bond is strengthened.

> The learning environment in family medicine, which emphasises patient-centredness, provides unique opportunities for learners to experience relationships that have developed over time.

Nurturing humanism in family medicine

Almost 100 years old, Francis Peabody's quote[1] outlines the essential ingredients of humanistic healthcare—showing interest, motivated by caring. A humanistic healer places the patient at the centre of their work. In contemporary medical education, teaching humanism does not require sophisticated equipment, but it does require protected curriculum time, thoughtful role modelling, and institutional commitment. A recent review on patient-centredness emphasised the need for alignment between the theory and practice of patient-centredness.[4] This is facilitated when students have opportunities to debrief on their experiences to develop "habits of humanism".[6] Without these opportunities, learners risk experiencing emotional dissonance between the stated aim of the curriculum (e.g. patient-centred care), and what happens in practice (e.g. system-centred care).

> Protecting time to discuss relationships, their ups and downs, helps learners appreciate the bidirectional nature of humanistic healthcare.

Case Example 1

To illustrate how busy family doctors can role model humanistic care in a clinical setting, we use a case vignette of George (Box 7.1). If the focus is solely on biomedical care in the consultation, the rationale for questions, behaviour, and decisions made from a humanistic perspective may be unclear. Just as physicians justify prescribing decisions, in-depth explanation of humanistic communication skills, their interpretation, and consequent decision-making helps learners understand the praxis of humanism as a skill.

> Students need to understand how FM doctors bring humanism into their decision-making.

How is humanism currently understood in Asian medical schools?

Owing to globalisation, doctors in FM encounter more culturally diverse patients today. When providing care to a multicultural society, better intercultural understanding, humanistic values, and communication between doctors and patients are needed.[7] Ensuring safe and quality healthcare for all patients also requires doctors to understand how each patient's sociocultural and economic background affect their health beliefs, behaviours, values, and attitudes.[8] This has underscored the need for doctors in multi-ethnic countries, as in Asia, to be cognisant of their own communication skills and humanistic qualities and how these can impact patient-centred care.[9–12]

> Quality healthcare requires doctors to understand how sociocultural, economic, and spiritual backgrounds influence each patient's health beliefs.

In a family practice in Asia, patients, together with their families, bring with them their own perspectives of health and illness, and values to the healthcare system, which may differ from those of mainstream Western medicine. Their

BOX 7.1 GEORGE'S VISIT AND EXAMPLE OF A FACILITATED DEBRIEF

George is a 78-year-old man who attends healthcare regularly. He has diabetes and ischaemic heart disease. He is widowed and lives alone, in a two-room apartment, with limited income. Today, George's HBA1c is raised at 8.8. You open the visit by asking him about his hobby, card playing. You address his diabetes after some "small talk". When George vehemently declines an offer to see the dietician or change his medications, you are agreeable.

Domain of humanistic care	Teaching and learning activity	Rationale	Illustrated example
Integrity	Share a moment	Valuing people demonstrates care by exemplifying small acts of kindness[13]	Asking about a game of cards and listening to the answer
Excellence in holistic care	Use a bio– psycho– sociocultural approach	Identify the interplay of factors impacting a single visit	*Biomedical issues*—knowledge of guidelines, and multimorbidity *Psychological issues*—mood *Social concerns*—income, isolation, health literacy
Compassion	Cultivate curiosity	Use questions to promote perspective taking	What is it like to be George? What matters to George? What worries George?
Altruism	Role model attentive listening	Non-verbal cues are often subtle	Sharing your interpretation of these cues helps learners understand your actions; e.g. George didn't make good eye contact and was hesitant in his replies, answering in a less enthusiastic tone than usual
Respect	Promote self-reflection Bearing silent witness, acknowledging	Physician, patient, and student views may differ Being there can be as important as change	How did the visit make the learner feel? E.g.: Were they frustrated by George's lack of commitment to seeing the dietician or changing his medication?
Resilience	Celebrate the rewards of humanistic healthcare	Humanistic healthcare is a resource for a rewarding career and protects against burnout	Share the joy and inspiration of working with patients. When George agrees to change, it feels great!
Service	Think ahead— ask what will happen next?	Students are often exposed to episodic care, with few opportunities to anticipate patient follow-up	The physician may have a mental plan for follow-up to encourage increased social interaction

inability to understand, manage, and cope with illness or consequences of treatment frequently creates barriers to care, especially when compounded by differences between doctor and patient in language, literacy, socio-economic status, and cultural backgrounds.

Case Example 2

Insensitivity towards other people's cultures can cause awkwardness and misunderstanding in physician–patient communication and be misconstrued as being inhumane. A young medical student, speaking about the experiences she encountered while interviewing patients, said:

> "....sometimes when they say someone died in the family... in English we were taught to say, "sorry to hear that ... and all that. But in the Malay language ... it's culturally accepted if you don't say anything".

Cultural differences should not be viewed as differences in human beings, but rather as alternative ways of living and approaching life.

Case Example 3

In 2003, a study was conducted on "minority" groups of medical students in a FM clerkship in Hawaii where most of the students were Pacific Islanders and Asians. Students wrote a reflective report about illnesses experienced in their own families. Portraying their family dynamics, outlining their families' beliefs about illness, and noting the influence of those beliefs on the course of their families' illness and treatment helped to inculcate in "minority" groups of medical students how to learn to find common ground between the influence of their families' values and their own views, in a process of acculturation in the practice of medicine.[11]

Conclusion

Humanistic dimensions of clinical care cannot be explicitly taught to medical students but rather can be infused longitudinally into daily practice and medical education. With good role modelling and ongoing feedback to students during their interactions with patients, both scientific knowledge and humane feelings can be inculcated together in the learning process in a safe environment such as FM.

References

1. Peabody FW. The care of the patient. J Am Med Assoc. 1927;88(12):877–82.
2. Gold Foundation. Definition of Humanism [Webpage]. Available from: https://www.gold-foundation.org/definition-of-humanism/ (Accessed 24 June 2002).
3. Martimianakis MAT, Michalec B, Lam J, Cartmill C, Taylor JS, Hafferty FW. Humanism, the hidden curriculum, and educational reform: A scoping review and thematic analysis. Acad Med. 2015;90(11):S5–S13.
4. Bansal A, Greenley S, Mitchell C, Park S, Shearn K, Reeve J. Optimising planned medical education strategies to develop learners' person-centredness: A realist review. Med Educ. 2022;56(5):489–503.
5. Hazrati H, Bigdeli S, Gavgani VZ, Soltani Arabshahi SK, Behshid M, Sohrabi Z. Humanism in clinical education: A mixed methods study on the experiences of clinical instructors in Iran. Philos Ethics Humanit Med. 2020;15(1):1–10.
6. Cohen LG, Sherif YA. Twelve tips on teaching and learning humanism in medical education. Med Teach. 2014;36(8):680–4.
7. Watermeyer J, Thwala Z, Beukes J. Medical terminology in intercultural health interactions. Health Commun. 2021;36(9):1115–24.
8. McQuaid EL, Landier W. Cultural issues in medication adherence: Disparities and directions. J Gen Intern Med. 2018;33(2):200–6.
9. Balint E. The possibilities of patient-centered medicine. J Royal Coll Gen Pract. 1969;17(82):269.
10. Mead N, Bower P. Patient-centredness: A conceptual framework and review of the empirical literature. Soc Sci Med. 2000;51(7):1087–110.
11. Chandratilake M, Nadarajah VD, Mohd Sani RMB. IMoCC: Measure of cultural competence among medical students in the Malaysian context. Med Teach. 2021;43(sup1):S53–S8.
12. Ho M-J, Gosselin K, Chandratilake M, Monrouxe LV, Rees CE. Taiwanese medical students' narratives of intercultural professionalism dilemmas: Exploring tensions between Western medicine and Taiwanese culture. Adv Health Sci Educ. 2017;22(2):429–45.
13. Gillespie H, Kelly M, Gormley G, King N, Gilliland D, Dornan T. How can tomorrow's doctors be more caring? A phenomenological investigation. Med Educ. 2018;52(10):1052–63.

What to aim for

Principles of curriculum design

Everyone can stay the same. It takes courage to change.

John Assaraf

8

Addressing population needs

Hassan Salah, Saeed Soliman, and Marie Andrades

SUMMARY OF KEY LEARNING POINTS

- Addressing population needs requires an extensive understanding of the population the medical school serves.
- Medical colleges have a social responsibility to the community as well as to the students and faculty.
- The country's community health issues should form the crux of the curricular content.
- The curriculum must address its students' needs through student engagement and interventions supporting health as well as learning.
- Faculty development is key to delivering a curriculum receptive to the needs of the population.
- Challenges of incorporating population needs into the curriculum can be addressed through advocacy and community, faculty, and student engagement.

Outlining the population needs of the country

Globally, the health needs of communities are transforming rapidly. Climate change is impacting dramatically on population health and the COVID-19 pandemic has widened health inequity. All these changes should be addressed by adapting health systems to minimise disparities and ensure priorities are recognised and met. It is important for the family medicine (FM) curriculum to rapidly adapt to population and health system needs.

The first recommended goal of the Carnegie Foundation for the Advancement of Teaching Investigation on Medical Education is to "Standardise learning outcomes and general competencies and provide options for customising the learning process, providing opportunities for experiences in research, policy making, education, etc., reflecting the broad role played by physicians".[1] The health system–based curriculum emphasises

DOI: 10.1201/9781003325734-10

the need to "improve performance of the healthcare system in adapting core professional competencies into specific contexts, on the basis of global knowledge".[2]

The World Health Organisation (WHO) defines community health needs assessment as "a process that describes the state of health of local people; enables the identification of the major risk factors and causes of ill health; and enables the identification of the actions needed to address these risks". It is a continuous process of evolving and adapting health systems and medical curricula to readjust priorities and reallocate resources to minimise inequity in healthcare service delivery.[3]

> Medical schools' curricula must reflect the health needs of the catchment population they serve and must rapidly respond to change.

Population needs assessment must follow certain steps to include community, health systems, organisations, and other stakeholder's engagement[2] (Box 8.1).

The need for community-oriented primary care physicians

Primary care (PC) forms the essential base for a country's healthcare system. It functions as the most important service for maintaining a healthy population through disease screening, immunisation, health education, early detection, and prevention of disease. It fulfils the goal of universal health coverage (UHC). A robust PC reduces disease burden by improving community and population health.[4] The five principles of community-oriented primary care (COPC) are responsibility for (a) comprehensive care of a defined population; (b) care based on health needs and its determinants; (c) prioritisation of those needs to implement health programmes; (d) ensuring programmes integrate promotion, prevention, and treatment; and (e) community participation.[5]

PC physicians form the backbone of a country's healthcare system. They focus on integrating assessed population needs into healthcare delivery. In many countries, physicians graduate from medical school curricula which are entirely hospital based. They enter FM practice without any further training or orientation to the community they intend to serve. This creates a disconnect with the community needs and reduces the effectiveness of the care they provide.

PC physicians trained through community-oriented medical curricula focus not only on the patient but can also diagnose and manage based on the local

---

BOX 8.1 STEPS REQUIRED TO IDENTIFY POPULATION NEEDS[2]

- Profiling the population
- Deciding priorities
- Planning programmes (educational, public health, health systems) to address priorities
- Implementing planned programmes
- Evaluating programme impact

epidemiology of the disease.[6] They can explore the impact of the disease on the family, connecting it to the social determinants of health, and offer advice and intervention based on the population and public health picture. Offering holistic assessment and care to the patient, family, and community enhances disease prevention and health promotion. Evidence has clearly shown that countries with strong PC health systems have better health indicators than those without it.[7]

Inculcating PC concepts into the curriculum is essential to produce physicians responsive to population needs.

Population needs–based curricula: The role of PC education

Today's world is very distinct from the past. Climate change, increasing diversity, political enmity within regions and countries, all affect health. With rapid and changing modes of communication and interaction, people are more aware of their right to health and are vocal in expressing it. To be responsive to the population needs, the curriculum must be embedded in the community setting. This provides the base for experiential learning to recognise specific health issues within the relevant context and develop culturally, linguistically, and economically sensitive practice.[8]

Providing health needs assessment education is an essential element of undergraduate (UG) medical curricula. Using quantitative, qualitative, and comparative methods to determine the population's health problems requires community-based access to the population. This can only be achieved if medical schools invest in community-based teaching sites and clinics (Chapter 3).

A community-based curriculum addresses the social responsibility medical schools have towards population health.

Exploring medical school undergraduate and postgraduate curricula for their responsiveness to community needs

To introduce FM into the UG curriculum, adequate faculty numbers are required. Exploring the existing FM UG and postgraduate (PG) training programmes will not only address this need but also help scale up production of family physicians and strengthen family practice for UHC.[9]

Specific objectives include the following:

■ *Situation analysis:* Mapping and evaluating UG and PG FM educational programmes

■ *Demand-need analysis:* Comparing workforce production and community needs identifying any existing gaps in the availability of family physicians

■ *Action:* Proposing recommendations to scale up family physician training

Three main domains should be explored:

■ *Education:* The duration, content, and capacity for FM delivery in the curriculum. This is particularly important given the wide differences globally across medical schools. The presence of opportunities for continuous professional development in FM is crucial.

■ *Regulation:* The healthcare delivery systems, recognition and accreditation of training programmes, licensing procedures, granted privileges, and FM regulatory arrangements.

■ *Practice:* The family physicians' practice structures, employability, retention, remuneration, careers, and satisfaction etc.

Comprehensive survey of the country's existing FM educational programmes provides basic information needed for designing and implementing FM in the medical school curriculum.

Addressing students' learning needs

Needs assessment requires an assessment of the training and educational needs of individuals, groups, and organisations. Even though the curriculum developer may be an expert, to enhance student learning and ensure competencies are appropriate and achievable, the UG curriculum must align with the variance in students' backgrounds and needs. Interviews, focus groups, questionnaires, and Delphi methods are all appropriate needs assessment methods. It is important to synthesise information obtained in a logical, organised manner to ensure the formation of a learner-centred curriculum.

Students form the core users of the curriculum. Obtaining their views as consumers is critical to a responsive and dynamic FM curriculum.

Box 8.2 summarises the core learning outcomes a curriculum needs to address on population needs.

Faculty development

Community-based medical education is increasingly important within medical school curricula where faculty (who may not be trained FM doctors) supervise and support students to understand the population context when they see patients and families in community settings. This introduces a new skill set to be addressed in faculty development programmes.[10]

BOX 8.2 CORE ELEMENTS OF ADDRESSING POPULATION NEEDS

Should know:	The social determinants of disease
	The difference between disease presentation in a community versus hospital context
	The need for community-oriented medical schools
Should be able to:	Manage disease prevention and management within the community context
	Apply the knowledge of contributing factors within the community in prevention and management of disease
	Engage with the community for health promotion
Should be:	Responsive to the health needs of the community
	Empathetic and non-judgemental toward community norms and practices
	Willing to develop a mutually collaborative relationship with the community they serve

Specific elements of a faculty development programme for community-based teaching include:

■ *Setting expectations:* Awareness of the community ecosystem, including its sociocultural norms, resources, epidemiological patterns of disease, and health practices, is important. The local faculty should be inducted into the community-oriented curriculum.

■ *Inculcating adult learning principles:* Teachers need to instil lifelong adult learning within the learners.

■ *Incorporating FM as a core concept—developing clinical teaching skills:* In a busy FM practice setting with multiple learners, different education approaches may be needed, e.g. the 1-minute preceptor model,[11] SNAPPS (a six-step learner-centred teaching approach in outpatient settings).[12]

Enhancing constructive feedback skills: Mentoring students, often unfamiliar with the challenges of low socio-economic settings, is essential. Constructive reflection with feedback to set ongoing learning goals is important (Chapter 28).

Being cognisant of programme evaluation models: Faculty need to apply appropriate ones to evaluate their community teaching (Chapter 31).

Creating strategies for dealing with challenging learning situations: This can be essential given the complexity of enabling students to view patients holistically within the context of the local population—skills which may be very new to them.

Providing supportive mentorship: Faculty need training as mentors for community physicians and healthcare workers as well as students (Chapter 26).

Incorporating FM core concepts in faculty development (especially for those not trained as family doctors) is critical for effective curriculum delivery.

Tips for incorporating population needs into the curriculum

Sensitising medical education leaders

External and internal influences can play a major role in triggering the integration of FM into UG curricula.[13-15] Astute FM leaders can harness these to tip the balance towards PC education in the curriculum (Chapter 6).

External influences include health system demands, e.g. (i) government pressure for more PC physicians to ensure health provision for underprivileged populations; (ii) global medical workforce migration especially from developing to developed countries; (iii) medical curricular accreditation by international agencies stimulating change to meet global standards.

Internal influences include (i) a strong medical education department advocating reform to prepare students for the country's health needs; (ii) an overwhelming burden on tertiary care teaching hospitals where clinicians lack time to teach; and (iii) patient demand for care closer to home.

Identifying catchment communities

Medical schools are socially accountable to their communities (Chapter 3). Each school should identify its catchment community and provide services to improve local health indicators and systems. Important criteria for doing this are (i) geographical closeness to the medical school and attached teaching hospital(s); (ii) areas of deficient community resource; (iii) alignment of curriculum outcomes with community stakeholders' agendas for enhancing health; (iv) stakeholders' acceptance of student community placements; and (v) available physical infrastructure for students to brief and debrief.[16]

Developing community-based primary healthcare centres

Whereas some communities have established primary healthcare (PHC) centres to use for FM education, many have not. First, an open dialogue must be established with the community. Often the community can provide the physical infrastructure while the school offers human, technical, and material resources. Community members can become essential stakeholders in policy development to govern PHC centres and bring education onto the agenda.[14]

Ensuring student engagement

It is important to engage students in PHC policymaking processes and community education. This can be achieved by assigning students to families within the community to explore the social determinants of their health and build a sense of ownership of their patients' healthcare. Alternatively, students can conduct baseline community health needs surveys, evaluate the data, and implement PC intervention strategies. It is important to encourage students to develop PC research.[17]

Developing a responsive faculty

Developing a shared faculty vision of community-based PC education confirms their essential role and involvement in the process. Inducting FM doctors already practising within the community enhances motivation and involvement in curriculum implementation. Faculty development and opportunities for career progression prevent burnout. Adequate remuneration is necessary for faculty based in the medical school and for travelling to teaching medical students at community sites. Faculty provide important positive role models for students. Demotivated faculty can derail the entire curriculum if students see them as negative role models—an impression which is difficult to reverse.[18]

Conclusion

An UG medical school curriculum, responsive to local population health needs, ensures all students graduate as competent and sensitised physicians able to understand and practise within the whole context of their health system whatever specialty they subsequently enter.

References

1. Irby DM, Cooke M, O'Brien BC. Calls for reform of medical education by the Carnegie Foundation for the Advancement of Teaching: 1910 and 2010. Acad Med. 2010;85(2):220–7.
2. Quintero GA. Medical education and the healthcare system: Why does the curriculum need to be reformed? BMC Med. 2014;12(1):213.
3. Organization WH. Community Health Needs Assessment: An introductory guide for the family health nurse in Europe. Copenhagen; 2001. Report No.: 9289011947.
4. Schwarz D, Duong D, Adam C, Awoonor-Williams JK, Back D, Bang A, et al. Primary care 2030: Creating an enabling ecosystem for disruptive primary care models to achieve universal health coverage in low- and middle-income countries. Ann Glob Health. 2020;86(1):9.
5. Atun R. What are the advantages and disadvantages of restructuring a health care system to be more focused on primary care services? WHO Regional Office for Europe Health Evidence Network Report; 2004.
6. Sanyoto DVT, Syah NA. The role of primary care physicians (DLP) in community care. Rev Prim Care Pract Educ. 2018;1(1):3–5.
7. Starfield B, Shi L, Macinko J. Contribution of primary care to health systems and health. Milbank Q. 2005;83(3):457–502.
8. Gouda EM, Youssef WT. Needs assessment of the undergraduate medical students to incorporate courses on medical education into the undergraduate curriculum at the Faculty of Medicine, Suez Canal University. Intellect Prop Rights Open Access. 2014;2(1):100109.
9. Salah H, Kidd M. Family practice in the Eastern Mediterranean region universal health coverage and quality primary care. Boca Raton, FL: Taylor & Francis; 2019.
10. Langlois JP, Thach SB. Bringing faculty development to community-based preceptors. Acad Med. 2003;78(2):150–55.
11. Neher JO, Gordon KC, Meyer B, Stevens N. A five-step "Microskills" model of clinical teaching. J Am Board Fam Pract. 1992;5(4):419–24.

12. Wolpaw TM, Wolpaw DR, Papp KK. SNAPPS: A learner-centered model for outpatient education. Acad Med. 2003;78(9):893–8.

13. Hays R. Community-oriented medical education. Teach Teach Educ. 2007;23(3):286–93.

14. Wagdy T, Ladhani Z. Community based education in health professions global perspectives. Cairo, Egypt: The Eastern Mediterranean Regional Office of the World Health Organization; 2013.

15. Howe A. Twelve tips for community-based medical education. Med Teach. 2002;24(1):9–12.

16. Macharia PM, Ray N, Giorgi E, Okiro EA, Snow RW. Defining service catchment areas in low-resource settings. BMJ Global Health. 2021;6(7):e006381.

17. Pearson DJ, Lucas BJ. Engagement and opportunity in clinical learning: Findings from a case study in primary care. Med Teach. 2011;33(12):e670–e7.

18. Zelek B, Goertzen J. A model for faculty engagement in distributed medical education: Crafting a paddle. Can Med Educ J. 2018;9(1):e68–e73.

9

Addressing patient and family needs

Maria Sofia Cuba-Fuentes and Carmen Cabezas Escobar

SUMMARY OF KEY LEARNING POINTS

- Students need to approach patients, understanding that the disease, person, and the environment are not independent. A holistic approach to patient needs is essential.

- Addressing persons and family health needs is fundamental to curriculum design and should be incorporated across all years and specialties. It is not a course on its own.

- Students need communication skills training to learn to explore a person's life story narrative and understand their needs in the context of their social context and health.

- Values-based education is important enabling students to approach patients with sensitivity addressing their cultural, spiritual needs, and ensuring equality diversity inclusion.

- Family medicine (FM) placements enable students to see patients in family and social contexts and should be designed for longitudinal continuity of contact where possible.

Introduction

Person-centred medicine has long been described and supported by FM literature. It was considered as one of the six aims of quality by the National Academy of Medicine (USA).[1] Regardless of the clinical specialty, person-centred care (PCC) has been recognised as intrinsic to patient care. It is now the foundation of teaching about clinical care and communication across the medical school curriculum.

Simply speaking, patient-centred care medical education can be defined as being *about* the patients, *with* the patients, and *for* the patients, to ensure current and future doctors remain sensitive to all of the needs of the people they care for in their future careers regardless of specialty.[2] It is fundamental to the generalist skills all medical students should be competent in when they graduate from medical school.

DOI: 10.1201/9781003325734-11

Learning to be person-centred

It is impossible to practise medicine or care for people's health effectively without attention to the range of psychological and social issues embedded in the lives of all human beings. Medical students begin their undergraduate medical education with a superficial understanding of PCC. They recognise the need to listen and work collaboratively with the patient to plan their care. However, the skills needed for PCC must be explicitly integrated into the medical school curriculum for students to gain an in-depth understanding of, and become competent in, applying these principles to their clinical practice[3] (Chapter 22).

> Patient-centred care and enabling students to listen and work collaboratively with patients have become intrinsic to medical school curricula globally.

Traditionally, in the Flexner model (Chapter 11), basic science and the pathology and clinical presentations of diseases have been the starting point for learning to approach the patient. The curriculum emphasised how to take a correct medical history, carry out a proper physical examination, and then interpret laboratory tests. While this approach may ultimately lead the doctor to the correct medical diagnosis, the treatment plan would be incomplete without the exploration of the patient's life story narrative from which to build an understanding of their underlying illness and health.[4]

Understanding patients holistically in their personal and family social contexts and exploring the meaning that the disease has in both their personal and their families' lives are essential to reach a treatment plan based on shared decision-making. This empowers the patient to be a key participant in their care. Evidence shows it improves their experience with the healthcare provider, builds trust in the medical system, and results in better adherence to treatment[5] (Chapter 22).

> Understanding patients holistically by exploring their presenting complaint in the context of their personal and social life story builds trust and improves adherence to treatment.

Patient-centred clinical method

Stewart et al., acknowledging that the existing doctor-centred paradigm did not address patients' needs, developed the person-centred clinical method.[6] This clinical method is based on four components health professionals should address when they approach patients:

- *Address* the illness, health and disease
- *Approach* the person as a whole
- *Reach* a common agreement based on the definition of problems, objectives, and roles
- *Develop* the doctor–patient relationship[7,8]

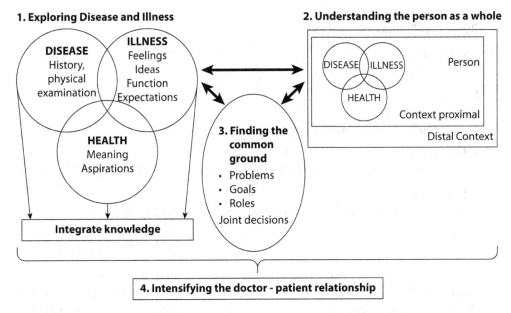

FIGURE 9.1 The person-centred method.[6]
Adapted from Stewart et al. (2014).

The first and the second components are especially important when addressing person and family needs (Figure 9.1).

Addressing illness, disease, and health

Traditionally, in the past, medical schools focused curriculum design on learning outcomes centred on students becoming experts in diseases common to a single specialty or discipline. Fortunately, there has been increasing recognition that with changes in population needs, such as ageing and increasing comorbidity (Chapter 8), this approach is no longer appropriate. Patients do not fit neatly into disease "boxes".

> The increasing complexity of healthcare as population needs change requires an understanding of patients' presentations in the context of illness and health, not only disease.

Based on Stewart et al.'s modelling, the biomedical approach to illness needs to be re-examined to be inclusive of patient and family needs. Students must be trained to explore the patient's narrative around illness and health as well as disease. The person's feelings around their ideas, expectations, and fears become of paramount importance to understand how an illness can impact on and alter the way a person functions. This approach needs to be built into the complete clinical encounter. Understanding the impact of the illness on a patient and their family could change the approach to the health problem (Box 9.1) (Chapter 22).

BOX 9.1 EXPLORATION OF ILLNESS

F: Feelings
How is that problem making you feel?

I: Ideas
What do you think is causing the problem?
What do you think could improve the problem

F: Function
Is the problem affecting your job or your daily routine?

E: Expectations
What do you expect from our consultation? How do you think I can help you?

Developing an understanding of a patient's needs relating to health may involve sensitively exploring personal values such as spirituality, cultural expectations, and the course of life events. Integrating communication training into the course for students to develop active listening skills, demonstrate empathy, etc. is essential and is explored in Chapter 22. Students should learn to understand the social determinants of health and patients' needs within the family context, the community, the available social support, and the local health system. Equality, diversity, and inclusion are values being progressively inculcated into medical institutions globally.

Health must be thought of as a concept unique to each person that goes beyond the absence of disease. It can encompass the aspirations and aims of every patient. People can have values and ways of seeing the world from a completely different perspective from the health professional caring for them.[9] Instilling the concept of value-based healthcare to enable students to understand, and be sensitive to, views and prejudices different from their own is gaining recognition and importance in medical education (Chapter 12).

> Patients can see the world in diverse ways often very different from the health professionals perspective. Respecting this and addressing equality, diversity, and inclusion is important.

Health is better explored in a continuous relationship between doctor and patient. Students, on short placements, must be encouraged to explore the significance of health for a person in a single medical encounter. However, the increasing introduction of longitudinal integrated clerkships (Chapter 17) is designed to enable students to explore and follow patients and their families' needs as they journey though the health system.

Addressing families in the clinical encounter

In many cultures, families are the principal health resource for an individual. They take care of a family member when they become acutely ill, disabled, or develop a chronic condition. To gain a better clinical approach to health problems, exploring the family perspective is essential. It is important that the approach to a family is inclusive, highly contextual, and culturally sensitive acknowledging different patterns of socialisation, gender, sexuality, religious practices, etc.[8] By exploring the roles of different individuals in the family, how they interact, and their strengths and weaknesses, students can build an understanding of how the patient faces up to and deals with healthcare issues.

The definition of family can range from one that is traditional to one that may include close friends and caregivers whom a patient regards as their family. Students must approach the family as an open social system and be aware of the integral and systemic conception of health, illness, and disease as a social product. As healthcare becomes more holistic, culturally diverse, and collaborative, assessing patient and family needs becomes increasingly necessary. Students should be encouraged to explore the family context and influences in the clinic, on home visits and through inpatient care. Introducing early clinical exposure (Chapter 15) and designing longitudinal attachments on FM placements (Chapter 17) are increasingly important innovations in medical education. This helps students, often from very different social backgrounds, to develop an understanding of health behaviours, their influence on patient management, and how protective mechanisms when dealing with disease can be developed.

> Respectful, culturally aware communication with patients and their families needs to be learnt, reflected on, supported, and continuously practised by students on FM placements.

Encouraging students to be family-centred does not undermine the role of the individual in making their decisions. Rather, it insists that medical care must be contextualised in the patient's life experiences. The role of the family and its different members in the planning of care at home must be recognised. As healthcare moves to increasingly involve patients in their healthcare, emphasising the needs of patients and their families is gaining increasing status in medical education. The development of health advocacy roles for health issues, including health promotion for individuals and their families, is a further benefit.

Family placements, and the generalist approach to healthcare, offer ideal and unique opportunities for students to explore and reflect on these issues. Improving the clinical environment for patients through listening and empathising with their lives concurrently improves the environment for learners.[10]

Shared decision-making

To learn how to make shared decisions with patients, students can be guided to define a list of problems in the encounter and then prioritise goals and treatment with the patient.[7] Elwyn et al. proposed a model based on introducing choice, discussing the options, and exploring the preferences before reaching a decision.[11] It is important for students to know that some patients require more than one meeting to make complex decisions in different contexts. The family's participation can play an important role in supporting these decisions. The importance of reaching shared decisions though cannot be underestimated. It is intrinsic to accomplishing kind, compassionate, and patient-centred healthcare.[12] How to achieve this is further explored in Chapter 22. As with all learning outcomes, it is essential that the skills needed for ensuring that communication is patient-centred must be explicitly assessed to avoid marginalisation as "soft" skills not intrinsic to everyday practice. The fifth section on assessment explores this in more depth.

> Explicitly assessing learning outcomes centred on patient-centred communication in the FM context of the family and community is essential for students to value its importance.

Conclusion

Future clinicians need to accomplish competences not only related to clinical diagnosis and management expertise. In a medical encounter, understanding the person as whole is both challenging and necessary. Medical students must understand how to holistically approach patients to establish their needs in the context of their families and community and then achieve shared decisions when agreeing their management.[13]

Assessing patients' and families' needs is an essential competence that future doctors need on graduation whatever their subsequent career. FM placements in the community with the patient's family, especially if designed for students to experience continuity of care, are increasingly important in achieving this.

References

1. Institute of Medicine (IOM). Crossing the quality chasm: A new health system for the 21st century. Washington, DC: National Academy Press; 2001. https://nam.edu/about-the-nam/
2. Baker A. Book: Crossing the quality chasm: A new health system for the 21st century. BMJ. 2001;323:1192. https://doi.org/10.1136/bmj.323.7322.1192
3. Hearn J, Dewji M, Stocker C, Simons G. Patient-centered medical education: A proposed definition. Med Teach. 2019;41(8):934–38. https://doi.org/10.1080/0142159X.2019.1597258
4. Henschen BL, Ryan ER, Evans DB, Truong A, Wayne DB, Bierman JA, et al. Perceptions of patient-centered care among first-year medical students. Teach Learn Med. 2019;31(1):26–33.
5. Lovo J. Ian McWhinney: The nine principles of family medicine. Arch Med Fam. 2021; 23(2):101–8.
6. Stewart M, Brown J, Weston W, McWhinney I, McWilliam C, Freeman T. Patient-centered medicine: Transforming the clinical method. Boca Raton, FL: CRC Press; 2014. p. 360.
7. Heredia Lima C, Juan José Rodríguez Lazo EsSalud Lima P, Guillermo Kaelin de la Fuente Lima P, Profesora P, Asistente M, Cuba-Fuentes M, et al. CONTRIBUCIÓN ESPECIAL/ SPECIAL CONTRIBUTION La medicina centrada en el paciente como método clínico Patient-centered medicine as a clinical method. 2016;50–9.

8. Membrillo A, Fernandez MA, Quiroz JR, Rodriguez JL. Familia. Introducción al estudio de sus elementos. Mexico: Editores de textos Mexicanos; 2008.

9. Cassell EJ. The nature of healing: The modern practice of medicine. Online ed. Oxford Academic; 2012. https://doi.org/10.1093/acprof:oso/9780195369052.001.0001

10. Philibert I, Patow C, Cichon J. Incorporating patient- and family-centered care into resident education: Approaches, benefits, and challenges. J Grad Med Educ. 2011;3(2):272–78.

11. Elwyn G, Frosch D, Thomson R, Joseph-Williams N, Lloyd A, Kinnersley P, et al. Shared decision making: A model for clinical practice. J Gen Intern Med. 2012;27(10):1361–67.

12. Málaga G, Romero ZO, Málaga AS, Cuba-Fuentes S. Shared decision making and the promise of a respectful and equitable healthcare system in Peru. Z Evid Fortbild Qual Gesundhwes. 2017;123–124:81–4. Available from: http://dx.doi.org/10.1016/j.zefq.2017.05.021

13. Cuba MS, Campuzano J. Explorando la salud, la dolencia y la enfermedad. Rev Medica Hered. 2017;28(2):116.

10

Competency-based curricula

Maria Michelle Hubinette and Marcelo Garcia-Dieguez

SUMMARY OF KEY LEARNING POINTS

- Competency-based education (CBE) sets predetermined competency outcomes which students must achieve to practise safely on graduation.
- Learners achieve competency at different rates. Compared to traditional time-dependent curricula, CBE recognises that time to achieving competency is flexible.
- The goals, structure, and content of CBE curricula must be defined to support progressive achievement of competencies, disciplinary integration, and whole-task learning.
- Faculty educators need training in coaching and mentoring skills to move from directive teaching methods and support student lifelong learning.
- Family medicine (FM) provides an important context for embedding generalism throughout an undergraduate medical school curriculum.

Defining competency-based education

Numerous definitions of competence exist[1]; the following one prioritises competence from an operational perspective and can be applied across different contexts: "Competence is one's ability to do the right thing at the right time, in the right way, in a specific complex professional context".[2]

CBE has, as its main focus, a set of predetermined outcomes which represent a description of what learners need to be able to do by graduation. CBE focuses more on the end goal of learning rather than on the content or process of learning. In CBE, the focus is on ensuring that graduates are prepared to face the challenges of practice on graduation. CBE and its components are defined as "a framework of outcome competencies, sequenced developmental progression,

DOI: 10.1201/9781003325734-12

tailored learning experiences, competency-focused instruction, and programmatic assessment".[3]

> Curricula based on CBE focus on students achieving the predetermined competencies they need to practise safely on graduation.

Despite significant criticisms and scepticism, CBE has been widely adopted. It is often considered the "best" way to prepare professionals for adequate and safe delivery of patient care.[4,5] Many competency frameworks have been developed to guide outcomes of postgraduate training, e.g. the CanMEDS Physician Competency Framework[6] and the Outcome Project of the Accreditation Council for Graduate Medical Education (ACGME).[7] Undergraduate education too has increasingly moved to CBE. Examples include the General Medical Council Outcomes for Graduates[8] and Competence-based Undergraduate Curriculum for the Indian Medical Graduate.[9] The College of Family Physicians of Canada has articulated a set of undergraduate competencies specific to FM.[10]

Competencies represent a description of what a learner (or physician) is capable of doing. Thus, in CBE, competencies should inform both curriculum and assessment. The opportunities that learners are given must support progress towards, and achievement of, the stated competencies. Some jurisdictions have used the concept of entrustable professional activities (EPAs)[11] to describe units of professional work that could be entrusted to a graduate once they have achieved and demonstrated competence. It is claimed EPAs operationalise competencies and facilitate curricular implementation and assessment.[12]

Given its focus on outcomes rather than time or process, CBE demands more flexible training time, to allow trainees to achieve the expected outcomes. Learners will progress towards competence at different rates and with various degrees of support. This differs from traditional time-based education where learners were assumed to have obtained the required knowledge and skills based on the length of time spent. CBE implies the need to explore assessment models that better reflect and make evident development of expected competencies (Chapter 27).

> In contrast to traditional time-based education, CBE acknowledges that learners achieve competency at different rates with varying levels of support.

Competency-based curricula

Curriculum CBE planners need to define and design the goals, structure, and content of the curriculum to support progressive achievement of the competencies expected of the graduate to practise safely in the workplace. The focus of a competency-based curriculum (CBC) is a defined set of learning outcomes or competencies. The goal is the learner's achievement of these competencies. The structure should be flexible in time and learning opportunities reflecting differential trainee progress towards competency.

The curriculum should promote disciplinary integration[13] as competencies are, by their very nature, integrated (Chapter 11). Each professional competency integrates knowledge, skills, and approaches from, or relevant to, different disciplines. The content is delivered via engagement in relevant, whole–task learning opportunities, an approach that mirrors the concept of EPAs which centre on real tasks and scenarios in authentic contexts.[14] It uses tasks as curricular sequence organisers and provides students with a variety of learning tools to achieve the progressive mastery of these tasks.

> Students need to integrate the relevant knowledge, skills, and attitudes to achieve competence in complex professional tasks. CBC structure needs disciplinary integration and whole-task learning.

CBCs should include learners as active participants in learning and assessment promoting a learner-centred approach to foster differential progression. Teachers' roles as coaches and role models are critical in competence development; faculty development is crucial to prepare teachers for these roles (Chapter 26).

The multidimensional characteristics of competencies require the use of an assessment model based on formative assessments in different contexts and from different observers. This programmatic approach is addressed in Chapter 27. It informs learners and teachers of competence development allowing for high-stakes decisions on completing a training phase.[15] It enables struggling students to be identified and supported (Chapter 30). This model, based on authentic workplace assessment, fits better with the CBE concept and reflects the uncertainty of real-world healthcare.[15]

Table 10.1 compares the main characteristics of time-based ("traditional") and competency-based curricula.[16]

TABLE 10.1 Main characteristics of time-based and competency-based curricula[16]

Curriculum aspects	Time-based	Competency-based
Structure	Discipline based, linear, fixed sequence	Integrated, flexible, electives
Focus	Content	Outcomes
Content	Encyclopaedic approach	Relevant, paced, whole-task learning
Goal	Knowledge acquisition	Demonstration of competence, lifelong learning skills, knowledge and skills application
Actors	Teacher-centred Teacher as lecturer	Student-centred Teachers as role models and coaches
Assessment	Retrospective knowledge acquisition verification Norm referenced, summative	Programmatic assessment (portfolio, work-based assessment) Criterion referenced, formative
Programme completion	Fixed time	Variable time

Faculty development is essential to prepare teachers for new roles as coaches and role models for formative assessment and student–centred lifelong learning.

The added value of FM and generalism

Generalism can be defined as "a philosophy of care … distinguished by a commitment to the breadth of practice within each discipline and collaboration with the larger health care team to respond to patient and community needs".[17] This is in stark contrast to increasing specialisation. The full implications for future healthcare delivery are fully covered in Chapter 1. It is imperative that generalist principles are embedded through CBE in the education of all physicians, regardless of ultimate specialty choice.[18] In the undergraduate context, to ensure that generalism is embedded throughout the curriculum and aligned with assessment, the competencies should reflect a holistic generalism perspective, representing broad, undifferentiated skills and abilities that set learners up for success in any specialty, including FM.[19,20] The goals, structure, and content of the undergraduate CBE curriculum must embody and reflect principles of generalism. Table 10.2 outlines features of CBE curricula grounded in generalism.

Key generalism principles (e.g. complexity, continuity of care, context and adaptive expertise, and coordination of care) are summarised in Table 10.3 and explored in detail throughout this book. For example, *comprehensiveness* can be defined as care that encompasses the whole person rather than just the disease.[19,20] Comprehensive care is less about treating the disease and more about well-being and daily functioning, ensuring a holistic understanding of illness from the patient's perspective to encompass prevention, cure, and/or palliation across the life cycle. (Chapter 9). Competency in comprehensiveness covers exploring undifferentiated

TABLE 10.2 Main characteristics of FM/generalist competency-based curriculum[16]

Curriculum aspects	Competency-based FM/generalist curriculum
Structure	Integrated flexible longitudinal Focus on continuity and coordination of care
Outcomes	Focus on generalism, comprehensive care, community-responsiveness, adaptability
Content	Relevant, whole-task learning opportunities emphasising comprehensiveness, complexity, multimorbidity, and context
Goal	Achieving competence includes skills in lifelong learning, generalism orientation, and breadth of competence regardless of specialty
Actors	Student-centred Family physicians as leaders, role models, and coaches
Assessment	Programmatic assessment (portfolio, work-based assessment), criterion referenced Formative, with attention to context
Length	Variable time to completion

TABLE 10.3 Key principles of generalism translated to CBC

Principles	Description[19,20]	Examples of curricular opportunities[19]
Comprehensiveness	• Care of whole person rather than disease • Focus on well-being and daily functioning rather than treatment of disease • Create holistic understanding of illness from the patient's perspective • Goals of prevention, cure, and/or palliation across the life cycle • Undifferentiated symptoms unclassified by body system or disease[21] • Broad scope of practice	• Reduce the focus on making a diagnosis (e.g. in case-based learning) and consider patient care well beyond disease cure or treatment • Interaction with patients in generalist contexts provides opportunities to learn from patients with undifferentiated conditions, non-specific or unclassified symptoms, or a wide range of concerns
Complexity	• Management of multimorbidity and a complex interplay of medical and social factors rather than treating a single disease or condition in isolation of other diseases or conditions or without consideration of the context of the patient and care environment	• Explicitly teach about comorbid conditions and complexity rather than always teaching about diseases or conditions in isolation • Make explicit the interactions between conditions, additional morbidity and challenge with daily function, cost of treatments, potential medication interactions, etc.
Continuity of care	• Recurring connection between a doctor and patient over a period of time[21,26]. • Undifferentiated, unclassified symptoms evolve and manifest over time • Longitudinal care may reduce unnecessary investigations or treatment and enable personalised care to be tailored to patient needs	• Highlight benefits of continuity of care, including improved patient outcomes along with patient satisfaction, more opportunities for health promotion, improved treatment adherence, fewer hospitalisations, and reduced mortality[26] • Include longitudinal placements such as integrated clerkships or following a panel of patients over time to enhance continuity
Context expertise, adaptive expertise[27]	• No two patients' problems nor contexts are identical. There is often ambiguity and uncertainty in practice • Consider patient and practice context • Responding appropriately to inconstancy of context requires *adaptive expertise* (Chapter 23)	• Focus on application of knowledge tailored to the context and specific circumstances of individual patients, physical location, cultural context, available resources, etc.
Coordination of care	• An antidote to fragmentation of care • Coordination of care can occur across and between specialties, within and between organisations, and concerning medical and social aspects.[20] Coordination of care ensures that the big picture is maintained, and collaboration and teamwork promoted	• Sharing with learners how communication and collaboration happens and how teams of all configurations work together to provide care

symptoms to identify the problem, not just physical pathology but the broad illness experience. Patients may present early in their illness trajectory with undifferentiated symptoms unclassified by body system or disease. Regardless of specialty, comprehensiveness represents a broad scope of practice and a wide range of unspecified patients and undifferentiated issues.[19,20]

> Generalist FM-based outcomes address comprehensiveness, complexity, context and adaptive expertise, continuity, and coordination of care. FM is an ideal context for learning these.

Operationalising a family medicine competency-based curriculum

A complete curricular reform to address CBE, with or without the EPA concept, is a major institutional challenge. Table 10.3 offers examples of how the key principles of generalism can be operationalised into a CBC. There are many successful examples around the world.[21–24] The Argentinian experience illustrates the FM and generalism context.[24] The curricular design for the initial programme phase is organised around the individual and family life cycle. It incorporates the concept of community-oriented primary healthcare by giving the students the opportunity to interact with people in the community, analyse their health needs, and, guided by teachers, plan interventions to improve their situations.[24]

Evaluation to monitor progress throughout CBC reform is essential (Chapter 31). Schneider et al.[25] provide details about how a FM-specific CBC was introduced into the FM clerkship as their school underwent curricular renewal. Kelly et al.[19] have suggested ways in which teachers can reinforce concepts of FM during undergraduate curriculum.

Conclusion

CBE is focused on learner achievement of competence as defined by a set of competency-based learning outcomes. CBCs include opportunities for progressive achievement of competencies, integration of knowledge and skills from across broad disciplines, and authentic whole-task learning. A FM context is ideal for embedding generalist principles into the undergraduate curriculum.

References

1. Hodges B. Medical education and the maintenance of incompetence. Med Teach. 2006;28(8):690–96. doi: 10.1080/01421590601102964
2. Saucier D, Schipper S, Oandasan I, Donoff M, Iglar K, Wong E. Key concepts and definitions of competency-based education [PowerPoint presentation]. Mississauga, ON: College of Family Physicians of Canada. 2011. Available from: https://www.cfp.ca/content/cfp/58/6/707.full.pdf

3. Van Melle E, Frank JR, Holmboe ES, Dagnone D, Stockley D, Sherbino J. International competency-based medical education collaborators: A core components framework for evaluating implementation of competency-based medical education programs. Acad Med. 2019;94(7):1002–09. doi: 10.1097/ACM.0000000000002743

4. Morcke AM, Dornan T, Eika B. Outcome (competency) based education: An exploration of its origins, theoretical basis, and empirical evidence. Adv Health Sci Educ Theory Pract. 2013;18(4):851–63. doi: 10.1007/s10459-012-9405-9

5. Imanipour M, Ebadi A, Monadi Ziarat H, Mohammadi MM. The effect of competency-based education on clinical performance of health care providers: A systematic review and meta-analysis. Int J Nurs Pract. 2022;28(1):e13003. doi: 10.1111/ijn.13003

6. Frank JR, Danoff D. The CanMEDS initiative: Implementing an outcomes-based framework of physician competencies. Med Teach. 2007;29(7):642–47. doi: 1080/01421590701746983

7. Swing SR. The ACGME outcome project: Retrospective and prospective. Med Teach. 2007;29(7):648–54. doi: 10.1080/01421590701392903

8. General Medical Council. Outcomes for graduates. 2018. Available from: https://www.gmc-uk.org/-/media/documents/outcomes-for-graduates-2020_pdf-84622587.pdf?la=en&hash=35E569DEB208E71D666BA91CE58E5337CD569945 (Accessed 19 December 2022).

9. Medical Council of India. Competency based undergraduate curriculum for the Indian medical graduate. Vol. 1;2018. pp. 1–257.

10. The College of Family Physicians of Canada. Undergraduate competencies from the family medicine perspective. 2019. https://www.cfpc.ca/CFPC/media/Resources/Education/CanMEDS-FMU-2019_Final_EN.pdf (Accessed 19 December 2022).

11. Association of Faculties of Medicine of Canada (AFMC). Entrustable professional activities for the transition from medical school to residency. 2016. Available from: https://md.utoronto.ca/sites/default/files/afmc_entrustable_professional_activities_en.pdf

12. Ten Cate O, Taylor DR. The recommended description of an entrustable professional activity: AMEE guide no. 140. Med Teach. 2021;43(10):1106–14. doi: 10.1080/0142159X.2020.1838465

13. Harden RM. The integration ladder: A tool for curriculum planning and evaluation. Med Educ. 2000;34(7):551–7. doi: 10.1046/j.1365-2923.2000.00697.x

14. Vandewaetere M, Manhaeve D, Aertgeerts B, Clarebout G, Van Merriënboer JJ, Roex A. 4C/ID in medical education: How to design an educational program based on whole-task learning: AMEE guide no. 93. Med Teach. 2015;37(1):4–20. doi: 10.3109/0142159X.2014.928407.

15. Schuwirth L, van der Vleuten C, Durning SJ. What programmatic assessment in medical education can learn from healthcare. Perspect Med Educ. 2017;6(4):211–15. doi: 10.1007/s40037-017-0345-1.

16. Saucier D, Shaw E, Kerr J, Konkin J, Oandasan I, Organek AJ, Parsons E, Tannenbaum D, Walsh AE. Competency-based curriculum for family medicine. Can Fam Physician. 2012;58(6):707–8.

17. Royal College of Physicians and Surgeons of Canada. Report of the generalism and generalist task force. Ottawa, ON: Royal College of Physicians and Surgeons of Canada. 2013. Available from: https://www.royalcollege.ca/ca/en/educational-initiatives/educational-generalism-medical-education.html.

18. The Future of Medical Education in Canada (FMEC). A collective vision for MD education. The Association of Faculties of Medicine in Canada; 2010.

19. Kelly MA, Wicklum S, Hubinette M, Power L. The praxis of generalism in family medicine: Six concepts (6 Cs) to inform teaching. Can Fam Physician. 2021;67(10):786–88. doi: 10.46747/cfp.6710786

20. Nutik M, Woods NN, Moaveni A, Owen J, Gleberzon J, Alvi R, Freeman R. Assessing undergraduate medical education through a generalist lens. Can Fam Physician. 2021;67(5):357–63. doi: 10.46747/cfp.6705357

21. Kiguli-Malwadde E, Olapade-Olaopa EO, Kiguli S, Chen C, Sewankambo NK, Ogunniyi AO, Mukwaya S, Omaswa F. Competency-based medical education in two Sub-Saharan African medical schools. Adv Med Educ Pract. 2014;5:483–89. doi: 10.2147/AMEP.S68480

22. Ten Cate O, Graafmans L, Posthumus I, Welink L, van Dijk M. The EPA-based Utrecht undergraduate clinical curriculum: Development and implementation. Med Teach. 2018;40(5):506–13. doi: 10.1080/0142159X.2018.1435856

23. Maaz A, Hitzblech T, Arends P, Degel A, Ludwig S, Mossakowski A, Mothes R, Breckwoldt J, Peters H. Moving a mountain: Practical insights into mastering a major curriculum reform at a large European medical university. Med Teach. 2018;40(5):453–60. doi: 10.1080/01421590601102964

24. Saulino JC, Sánchez MN, Busaniche JN, Durante E, Schwartzman G. Planning of teaching activities in an integrated curriculum: The risk of "disintegration". Rev Hosp Ital B. Aires. 2020; 40(3):13. Available from: https://www1.hospitalitaliano.org.ar/educacion/revista/index.php?contenido=ver_articulo.php&id_articulo=114610&id_rev=187&datorev=Septiembre+2020+volumen+40+N%26uacute%3Bmero+3 (Accessed 13 May 2022).

25. Schneider B, Biagioli FE, Palmer R, O'Neill P, Robinson SC, Cantone RE. Design and implementation of a competency-based family medicine clerkship curriculum. Fam Med. 2019;51(3):234–40. doi: 10.22454/FamMed.2019.539833

26. Pereira Gray DJ, Sidaway-Lee K, White E, et al. Continuity of care with doctors: A matter of life and death? A systematic review of continuity of care and mortality. BMJ Open. 2018;8:e021161. doi: 10.1136/bmjopen-2017-021161

27. Mylopoulos M, Kulasegaram K, Woods NN. Developing the experts we need: Fostering adaptive expertise through education. J Eval Clin Pract. 2018;24(3):674–77. doi: 10.1111/jep.12905

11

Designing an integrated curriculum

Saima Iqbal and Val Wass

SUMMARY OF KEY LEARNING POINTS

- Developing an undergraduate (UG) integrated curriculum is an iterative process dependent on well-structured design and delivery.
- Structuring the curriculum to develop horizontal integration of theoretical basic science with practical clinical learning and vertical integration to build deeper learning is important.
- Aligning learning and contextualising FM in all assessment processes is essential to drive learning.
- Integrating FM into an UG curriculum requires a dedicated and committed team to champion the importance of primary care and the learning opportunities it offers.
- FM Faculty must be visible across all campus curriculum processes and be active role models whether delivering personal care, tutoring, mentoring, or as academic primary care researchers.

Introduction

The Astana Declaration of 2018 recognises the importance of strengthening primary healthcare for provision of Universal Health Coverage and ensuring high-quality care for all without undue financial burden. An integrated health system with primary care at its core and linked with community services is crucial for its implementation.[1] Strong evidence is emerging that exposure to family medicine (FM) at medical school is essential to understand the role of primary care in healthcare delivery and to open opportunities to learn generalist skills which are not readily available in the specialist hospital environments.

DOI: 10.1201/9781003325734-13

The challenge of changing traditional medical education

It is important to ask "why" the UG curriculum globally has been slow to change from the format established by Flexner a century ago in the United States and Canada.[2] Traditionally, learning has remained centralised in tertiary or secondary care centres. The exposure of medical students to primary care settings during medical school is limited, even in countries where FM is well established.[3] Yet, evidence is emerging that FM placements as an undergraduate can inspire students to train in FM.[4] In many low middle income countries (LMICs), primary care is less well developed in the community. There may be no FM faculty presence in the medical schools. Without these structures, change is even harder to achieve in the face of strong tertiary and secondary care dominance.

Ironically, some LMIC students then graduate without training for FM delivery but can set up as untrained general practitioners by default. Arguably, had they been exposed to FM in their formative UG years, they would consider a future career as a FM specialist,[3] taking pains to get the required postgraduate experience. Integrating an understanding of FM into the UG curriculum has become essential. With increasing specialisation of hospital services worldwide, FM has become an optimum environment for witnessing, and learning from, the generalist continuity of healthcare patients receive in their communities.

> When integrating FM into UG curricula, adapting to local contexts is important. Globally, structures for FM delivery and its recognition as a specialty vary, especially in LMICs.

Medical schools must reflect and reassess their UG courses to include and expand exposure to FM. The challenge is to integrate ways to do this across the curriculum in line with local healthcare resources. Given the wide range globally of FM delivery, this can vary widely. Healthcare is changing with a move away from specialty silo delivery to more system-based delivery in line with changing population needs (Chapter 8).[4] Frameworks or models for visualising and implementing integration to harness local opportunities have become of paramount importance.[5] We outline ways of enacting this in a series of steps.

Curriculum integration

Step 1: Defining generalist learning outcomes

The beauty of FM is that patients are perceived holistically as people with medical conditions within their psychosocial context. As argued in Chapter 1, all medical students, whatever specialty they subsequently train in, should graduate with the holistic generalist skills which underpin all patient care. Given the changing healthcare needs introduced by ageing populations, multimorbidity, migration, climate change, the COVID-19 pandemic, etc., defining learning in terms of the biomedical single disease-based model is no longer appropriate. Students need the competencies to address undifferentiated diagnosis, cultural awareness, the social determinants of health, and increasing health inequity alongside understanding the impact of disease. FM offers an ideal learning environment for developing many of these competencies.

To achieve this generalist lens, the curriculum needs to offer holistic perspectives at all levels, while at the same time addressing the biomedical learning intrinsic to disease management. This can be realised by carefully defining the competencies medical students should have on graduation and the learning outcomes needed to achieve these (Chapter 10). These may already be available nationally[6] or supported by international principles and standards.[7] FM at the same time opens avenues to integrate clinical learning with interprofessional education and teamwork[8] (Chapter 18).

> FM as a learning environment enables students to integrate holistic patient-centred socially orientated principles with the biomedical disease-based knowledge delivered on campus.

Step 2: The SPICES Model[9]

The SPICES model of educational strategies for curriculum development offers a useful overall structure for an integrated design.[9] The acronym SPICES stands for six themes: (i) student-centred, (ii) problem-based, (iii) integrated, (iv) community-based, (v) electives, and (vi) systematic. Harden suggests that when developing a curriculum from scratch, each of these themes should be emphasised and delivered as a continuum across the years moving away from the more traditional blocks of systems or specialty rotations.[9] FM within this curriculum model can fulfil most of these criteria. Students can develop a problem-oriented approach, view the patient holistically in the community, and systematically integrate their basic science learning on body systems recognising its importance. True holistic patient-centred care, as integrated in the SPICES model, lends itself well to role modelling in the community as opposed to specialty-based rotations in the hospital.

Step 3: Horizontal and vertical integration

Structuring integration across the curriculum means abandoning the separation of basic science from clinical learning, traditionally taught in isolation from each other within specialty disease-based boundaries. The curriculum needs frameworks to provide students with improved integrated learning and deeper understanding of the relevance of knowledge to clinical practice. Horizontal and vertical integration of individual subjects and specialties within the medical curriculum enables students to gain a holistic perspective. Family physicians are trained to perform their clinical reasoning based on approaches to patients' symptoms, epidemiology, and demographic factors (Chapter 21). Integrating the curriculum will help students develop this reasoning. Integration should be both horizontal and vertical.

> Horizontally, integration of basic science with clinical practice and restructuring teaching vertically as expertise develops builds competence sequentially and aids deeper learning.

Horizontal integration means fusion of subjects taught within the same academic year, for example, anatomy with biochemistry and physiology, to give students a holistic, realistic, not fragmented understanding of how the normal structure and functions of the human body work. It is a fundamental move away from the traditional subject-based delivery. Change can be challenging as departments may fear their subject matter is under threat. It requires strong collaboration between departments and faculties when designing the curriculum to enable students to learn by systems across the SPICE model themes if these are being applied.

Vertical integration requires the incorporation of theoretical basic and behavioural science learning with the practical clinical sciences and experiential learning. Through vertical integration, the basic sciences are taught in the context of clinical and professional practice and vice versa. This enables clinical teaching to refer to basic concepts such as normal human physiology or the pathology of disease. It is a fundamental move from the traditional Flexner model of delivering two years in pure basic science before clinical contact is established[2] (Figure 11.1). It promotes

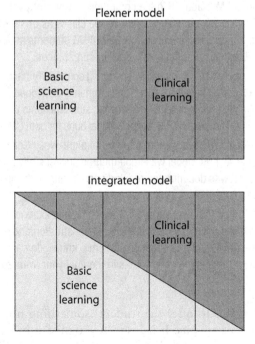

FIGURE 11.1 Comparing Flexnerian with Integrated curriculum modelling.

deeper situational learning built on situativity theory which enables knowledge, thinking, and learning to be situated (or located) in experience[10] (Chapter 19).

Step 4: The spiral curriculum

A final step is to build sequential deepening of learning as students progress through the course. A spiral curriculum[11] is one in which there is an iterative revisiting of subjects or themes from module to module. It is not simply the repetition of a topic but increasing the learning challenge of an encounter or task to build on previous ones and deepen the learning as the student moves cognitively along the novice to expert pathway (Figure 11.2).

Integrating FM into an UG curriculum is no mean feat. It requires a dedicated and committed team to become agents of change to champion the importance of primary care and the learning opportunities it offers. Faculty, staff, students, and administration officials all need clear shared deliverable goals defining the level of integration needed. Significant preparation and planning by all stakeholders are essential.

> Faculty must be active stakeholders in the preparation, planning, and delivery of a new integrated curriculum to champion primary care alongside secondary care.

We offer the strategic experience of embedding FM in the curriculum at Shifa College of Medicine, Islamabad, Pakistan:

1. We began by integrating clinical experience in FM with Community Medicine (CM), a basic science subject. This proved prudent as students then understood the relevance of CM learning to FM practised in the community. Family physicians were inducted into the CM department to set up community-based clinics as offshoots from the main hospital. These gave clinical exposure to Year 4 UG students and orientated them into community households and patients' social circumstances.
2. Once the clinics were functioning daily, conducting community-based research, an important CM curricular objective, became easier. The community developed a sense of trust with the FM services and were more receptive to allowing students home visits to conduct their research projects. The clinics became educational hubs for both CM and FM.
3. This partnership led to development of a formal eight-week Community and FM Clerkship in Year 4. This model was implemented successfully for several years. Student feedback was documented regularly confirming they valued participating in a FM-run primary care clinic.
4. Students highlighted that exposure to FM was a unique experience which made them feel like established doctors in real life. Once the institution and its hierarchy realised the importance of FM and its impact on students' knowledge and skills, FM was assigned its own Clerkship of nine weeks in the final year from 2022 onwards.

A valuable lesson was to offer the students something novel and not mimic the curricula of other departments. It helps to be cognisant of what is being taught in the other specialties and take a distinct route making the difference appreciable.

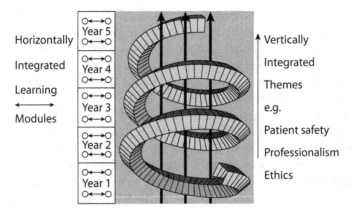

FIGURE 11.2 Horizontal and vertical integrated learning in a spiral curriculum.

While developing learning outcomes, the emphasis was on a holistic approach to dealing with common symptoms in different age groups, the biopsychosocial model of healthcare, patient-centeredness, and communication skills. Networking with other Family physicians practising in the community or in an Employee Health Clinic provided invaluable additional teaching sites for the FM Clerkship.

What are the benefits of integrated learning?

The benefits of integrating a curriculum are many. It helps tailor knowledge acquisition to the level needed for the clinical problem being addressed avoiding factual information overload, which can arise from traditional teaching by subject experts focused on their specialty alone. Linkages can be developed between concepts to heighten learning and improve understanding. Students from an integrated curriculum can see the end clinical goal and are motivated and more likely to be satisfied with their training. Integration enables clinical teachers to reflect on the scientific basis of practice and basic scientists to reflect on the clinical application of new knowledge and research. This promotes cooperation among different disciplines and prepares the students to become lifelong learners.

How to do it

The interpretation of the term "integration" may vary among different individuals. When developing an integrated curriculum for the first time, the steps and frameworks outlined above can prove invaluable. It is important to first identify what "depth" of integration is feasible. Even temporally aligning subjects into a common theme may prove to be challenging if the commitment is lacking, understanding of integrated teaching is limited, or the infrastructures to support it are not available. Significant time and effort are required for planning, organisation, and implementation. Institutions undertaking this process need to build staff member capacity. Faculty should fully understand the purpose and process of this intensive exercise. They must be made aware of their roles, responsibilities, and the challenges. It then involves developing study guides, case studies, and reference materials to be used in teaching and learning.

A curriculum committee or task force is usually given the mandate by the leadership to develop, organise, and implement the integrated curriculum. The committee may further subdivide itself or nominate subgroups to work on different aspects of curriculum development taking a lead for horizontal integration across a module or year(s) or to champion a vertical theme. It is important that both preclinical and clinical faculty are represented.

For FM to integrate, it is essential for its faculty to have their own teaching sites within, nearby, or at a distance from the tertiary care hospital. Ideally, there should be enough primary care sites with qualified family physicians so that students can witness and participate in how these services are delivered. This will require networking by FM faculty as well as an additional expense by institutions for travel and honoraria for doctors who are given the extra duty of clinical facilitation in a clinic.

> Networking with existing health services and incentivising their doctors into academic activities will pay off in the long run for development and strengthening of FM.

Assessment drives learning. This is an indisputable reality. The success of an integrated curriculum will depend on how well the assessment strategy is aligned and integrated with the intended learning outcomes and contextualised, where appropriate, within FM. Matching of the assessment method with the teaching modality is essential. The learning outcomes, teaching methodologies, and assessment strategies need to be communicated to, and delivered by, all stakeholders. It is essential the FM faculty is involved at all levels to ensure the assessments, whether written, workplace-based, or delivered as objective structured clinical examinations (OSCEs), give a clear message to students that their learning in FM is being tested (Chapters 27 and 29).

> It is crucial to accept that assessment drives learning. FM faculty must be active in developing and delivering all examinations to ensure students value learning in primary care.

Finally, the curriculum should be evaluated and revised in a timely fashion based on performance and feedback from students. This may even involve external review. It is important students see change in response to their feedback. For example, if a FM attachment has problems, then this must be addressed. Negative experiences of FM are difficult to reverse (Chapter 31).

The family physician as a role model

The Hippocratic oath commits every physician to pass on their knowledge and skills to future generations, yet there are very few trained family physicians who are academics (Chapter 5). In LMICs particularly, the family physician is often perceived as a doctor who will initially assess the patient and refer on to a specialist. The development and enhancement of FM as a specialty and the pressure being placed on its inclusion in UG curricula requires trained family physicians to act as role models, clinical tutors, faculty members, and researchers (Chapter 16).

> FM doctors at all levels of practice are crucial professional role models for students to both mirror values-based practice and inspire interest in FM as a career.

FM departments in teaching hospitals should collaborate with one another and share ideas about curriculum development and integration for the promotion and enhancement of their specialty. Family doctors as researchers are almost non-existent when compared to their clinician and basic scientist counterparts. Faculty members are in the best position to build their capacity in research methodology and contribute to the promotion of new knowledge in the field of health (Chapter 32).

References

1. Declaration of Astana and what it means for the global role of NAPCRG and WONCA. Ann Fam Med. 2020;18(2):189–90. doi: 10.1370/afm.2524.
2. Flexner A. Medical education in the United States and Canada: A report to the Carnegie Foundation for the Advancement of Teaching, 1910 bulletin no. 4. New York City: Carnegie Foundation for the Advancement of Teaching; 1910.
3. Amin M, Chandea S, Park S, Rosenthal J, Jones M. Do primary care placements influence career choice: What is the evidence? Educ Prim Care. 2018;29(2):64–7.
4. Bengoa R, Stout A, Scott B, McAlinden M, Taylor MA. Systems, not structures: Changing health and social care. 2016. Available from: https://www.health-ni.gov.uk/sites/default/files/publications/health/expert-panel-full-report.pdf
5. Breuer DG, Ferguson KJ. The integrated curriculum in medical education: AMEE Guide no. 96. Med Teach. 2015;37:312–22.
6. General Medical Council UK. Outcomes for graduates. 2020. Available from: https://www.gmc-uk.org/education/standards-guidance-and-curricula/standards-and-outcomes/outcomes-for-graduates/outcomes-for-graduates
7. World Federation for Medical Education (WFME). Basic medical education: WFME global standards for quality improvement. 2020. Available from: WFME-BME-Standards-2020.pdf
8. Strasser R, Berry S. Integrated clinical learning: Team teaching and team learning in primary care. Educ Prim Care. 2021;32(3):130–4. https://doi.org/10.1080/14739879.2021.1882886
9. Harden RM, Sowden S, Dunn WR. Educational strategies in curriculum development: The SPICES model. Med Educ. 1984;4:284–97.
10. Durning SJ, Artino AR. Situativity theory: A perspective on how participants and the environment can interact: AMEE Guide no. 52. Med Teach. 2011;33(3):188–99. https://doi.org/10.3109/0142159X.2011.550965
11. Harden RM, Stamper N. What is a spiral curriculum? Med Teach. 2009;21(2):141–3. https://doi.org/10.1080/01421599979752

12

Values-based education
Integrating professionalism into the curriculum

Kay Mohanna and Dinusha Perera

SUMMARY OF KEY LEARNING POINTS

■ Professionalism is a concept based on sociocultural values that are context specific.

■ Each institution should decide on its own definition.

■ Medical educators' expectations of professionalism should be clear and reflect the social contract between health professionals and the public.

■ Values-based practice (VBP) offers a framework for decision-making to form the foundation for a new way of teaching about professionalism.

■ FM educators can act as positive role models for medical students, demonstrating their professional values in action.

Defining professionalism

In health systems around the world, emphasis is placed on "professionalism" through codes of conduct for healthcare practitioners. It is a key element of curriculum design. Patients may find professionalism easy to define using layman's terms which might include "doing the right thing", "being trustworthy", and "being good at their job". It is, therefore, ironic that an international definition has proven hard to pin down despite a wealth of literature.[1]

The UK 2005 report on medical professionalism from the Royal College of Physicians (RCP) defined professionalism as "a set of values, behaviours and relationships that underpin the trust the public has in doctors".[2] More recently however, in 2018, the RCP concluded: 'There is increasingly a gap between what doctors are trained to do and the realities of modern practice'.[3] They abandoned the search for a revised definition and aimed to "explain, expand and interpret" the earlier definition.[3]

DOI: 10.1201/9781003325734-14

> Institutional professional standards must reflect the expectations of the patients and public.

In some regions of the world, the way the medical profession is viewed by patients and the public differs. In some cultures, it is still a hierarchical relationship and in others more egalitarian. Through a process of "democratisation of knowledge", information is increasingly not just in the hand of a privileged few, but available to all, via the internet and other sources. Definitions of professionalism that centre on the possession of expert knowledge are perhaps becoming less relevant.

Given these differences in sociocultural factors, perhaps it is not surprising that consensus on a generic, global definition of professionalism has not emerged. How to teach and assess professionalism, to ensure medical graduates achieve the high standards expected of them, should be contextualised to reflect the expectations and professional trust given to them by their institution and society.[4] Given these complexities, each teaching institution should agree with its own values and local definition to underpin learning about professional standards. This should inform their curricula on how to best teach, role model, and assess students.

Defining values

Defining professionalism to inform education and training can be challenging. The RCP definition importantly includes "values". Values are those principles which tend to determine a person's behaviour; principles which are "action-guiding", but which can mean different things to different people. Even the word "values" itself is hard to define. Sacket defined it as the "preferences, concerns and expectations" of individual patients[5] and, we might add, of practitioners.

> Values are action guiding but can mean different things to different people.

A crucial feature of both healthcare and healthcare education is that both are values-laden activities. Healthcare deals with often difficult and frequently emotional decision-making. Underlying values can be both complex (e.g. "best interests") and conflicting (e.g. incompatibility between the two values of "person-centred care" and "public health"). Citizens, healthcare professionals, and patients will hold a range of values as drivers for behaviours. These arise from their professional and personal codes, belief systems, experiences, and preferences. We define VBP as "a process that supports balanced decision making within a framework of shared values where complex and conflicting values are in play".[6]

Nurturing professionalism

In an attempt to "professionalise" physicians' behaviour, one response has been to increase regulatory measures of control such as revalidation and performance management.[7] This risks a negative, rules-based approach to professionalism and healthcare decision-making. It potentially achieves just the opposite, i.e., to "de-professionalise and erode trust".[8] The Indian Medical Council (Professional Conduct, Etiquette and Ethics) Regulations are currently under revision.[9] As Kane highlights: "a purely control-based regulatory response, as is being currently envisaged by the Parliament and the Supreme Court of India, runs the risk of undermining the trusting, interpersonal relations between doctors and their patients".[9]

Medical schools face a similar dilemma. A punitive or regulatory approach, focusing on fitness to practise in the undergraduate curriculum, fosters a negative view of professionalism. There is a risk, it sends a message to medical students that professionalism means "staying out of trouble" or, worse still, "not getting caught". Medical educators should nurture a positive view of professionalism, why it matters, and how it benefits future patients and society. Professionalism should be explicitly dissociated from increasing regulation and managerial oversight. Innovations in undergraduate curricula such as elements of reward or commendation for excellence, perhaps in activities that extend outside the taught components and beyond the assessed components, attempt to redress this.

> A positive approach to professionalism is important to foster excellence.

The impact of the null (or hidden) curriculum, or the unintended learning experiences, (Chapter 13) particularly in the clinical setting, underlines the importance of ensuring that our espoused values are aligned with the behaviours that are rewarded, to avoid negative role models for our students in the workplace. We must help our students develop the tools to continue to monitor and develop professionalism in both themselves and others. Students need the skills to reflect on what they see in practice and respond to situations where behaviours are falling below expected standards. Empowering students to speak up on behalf of patients if they observe actions raising patient safety concerns is crucial. Approaches can include reflective writing after clinical encounters, encouragement to document learning events, and the skill and confidence to open "courageous conversations".[10]

> Defining and role modelling professionalism should take place in all medical schools. Values-based practice offers a good platform for achieving this.

Values-based practice

Consider the role of the FM doctor, who takes pride in the role of advocate for her patient. Advocacy is one of the guiding principles (or values) that generalists use, helping to signpost a patient through the mass of medical uncertainty (Chapter 24). They aim to help make sense of a patient's symptoms, explain the options, and mutually develop a plan of action. The enactment of professionalism, in this context, does not require a list of preferred (or "right") outcomes, or adherence to rules, but a flexible process through which the family physician helps the patient make decisions that "fit" with the way they see the world. An important element of the model of VBP is that of *dissensus*: Differences in values are explored and acknowledged but are not necessarily "merged" or agreed upon, as they would in a consensus-building model. We can think of medical professionalism in FM as the competence of being able to explore and balance the three value domains of the patient, medical science, and our own personal ones.

> Advocacy is a guiding principle that generalists use, helping to signpost a patient through the mass of medical uncertainty.

Exploring global values

In May 2021, we asked around 50 colleagues across South Asia and the UK to list those aspects of professionalism they felt are important in graduating doctors. Our respondents were experienced trainers, workplace-based assessors, and examiners— all in active FM practice. It was not a scientific survey; more the email equivalent of a chat over coffee. Box 12.1 summarises the aspects where agreement emerged.

Whilst these core aspects of professionalism were similar, Box 12.2 shows that some differences were seen that may arise from differences in social

---

BOX 12.1 CORE ELEMENTS OF PROFESSIONALISM SHARED BY FM DOCTORS ACROSS SOUTH ASIA AND THE UK

Aspects of professionalism that graduates

Should know:	That community epidemiology of disease is different from hospital
	The limits of their knowledge and skills
	How to coordinate and oversee care within a team
	How generalist and specialist care fit together
	The importance of advocacy
	The importance of data management
	Financial and managerial aspects of healthcare provision
Should be able to:	Act in the best interests of the patient in front of them
	Solve problems
	Balance "today's conversation" with future decision-making with the patient
	Listen to the patient using "ears, eyes and heart"
	Engage in population-based health systems development
Should be:	Curious and interested in the patient
	Able to change—themselves, their approach, their systems
	Creative, imaginative leaders and owners of decisions
	Aware of the importance of creating a collaborative culture

BOX 12.2 AREAS OF VALUES-BASED DISSENSUS BETWEEN FM DOCTORS ACROSS SOUTH ASIA AND THE UK

UK FM doctors	South Asian FM doctors
The importance of work–life balance and knowing when to say no	Being the best or "never fail" approach
Person-centred decision-making	Rules-based decision-making
Equality between patient and doctor	Hierarchical culture, doctor expected to know
Primacy of patients in decision-making	Tendency towards doctors leading decisions
Individualism in decision-making	Collectivism in decision-making, e.g. family involvement

context. FM doctors described some elements of professionalism that are expressed differently in their communities. There was a recognition that some of these elements are in a state of flux as healthcare systems develop. The VBP model requires us to keep such differences in values visible and unsilenced, so that they can be taken into account.

Represented by the two columns in Box 12.2 are expressions of values that should be considered to exist to a greater or lesser extent in all doctors and all citizens; both doctors and patients will sit somewhere on a spectrum between the two positions. It seems likely that individual doctor–patient relationships will negotiate a way between the two positions depending on the individual values in play in that particular doctor–patient dyad, for any specific decision being considered. Perhaps there is, in fact, only one element of professionalism, the ability to recognise and respond creatively and imaginatively to such differences in values?

Many values are shared but differences arise and must not be lost across different contexts.

Teaching professionalism

From our discussions with FM colleagues, trainees, and trainers, we have developed five tips for teaching values-based professionalism in the undergraduate curriculum.

1. *Fostering debate:* Tutors have a responsibility to create a climate that fosters debate about differences in value. This encourages discussion and exchange of ideas and develops an understanding that there may be more than one appropriate course of action.

2. *Time, space, and emotional support* from tutors is needed to encourage learners to reflect on personal motivating values. This might be a new activity for students used to "finding out the right answer".

3. *Exploring complex and conflicting values:* The emphasis on "doing the right thing" in training should shift to a focus on developing "imaginative professionals" with the ability to explore complex and conflicting values.

4. *Critical reflection*, such as in learning logs or diaries, should be encouraged as a "safe space" to explore personal views and reactions to clinical challenges.

5. *VBP* should be considered an ongoing approach to developing professionalism and professional practice in medical school and beyond.

Conclusion

Professionalism is arguably one of the hardest elements to explicitly include in the undergraduate medical curriculum. It is largely based on sociocultural values and is the foundation of trust and expectations between society and its healthcare professionals. There is a lack of international consensus on its formal definition. Medical educators need to nurture the positive aspects of professionalism and develop standards appropriate for their society's context along with a mechanism to teach and role model positive behaviours. FM doctors have an important role in enabling students to explore complex and conflicting values in the generalist setting through reflective practice. Students should be encouraged to understand adherence to excellence in professionalism and its positive impact on the medical profession and its role in society.

References

1. O'Sullivan H, van Mook W, Fewtrell R, Wass V. Integrating professionalism into the curriculum: AMEE Guide no. 61. Med Teach. 2012;34:e64–e77.

2. Royal College of Physicians. Doctors in society: Medical professionalism in a changing world. London UK; 2005. https://shop.rcplondon.ac.uk/products/doctors-in-society-medical-professionalism-in-a-changing-world?variant=6337443013

3. Tweedie J, Hordern J, Dacre J. Advancing medical professionalism. London UK: Royal College of Physicians; 2018. https://www.rcplondon.ac.uk/projects/outputs/advancing-medical-professionalism

4. Cruess SR, Cruess RL. Professionalism: A contract between medicine and society. Can Med Assoc J. 2000;162(5):668–69.

5. Sacket DL, Straus SE, Scott Richardson W, Rosenberg W, Haynes RB. How to practice and teach EBM. 2nd ed. Edinburgh and London: Churchill Livingstone; 2000.

6. Fulford KWM, Peile E, Caroll H. Essential values-based practice. Cambridge: Cambridge University Press; 2021.

7. General Medical Council UK. Professional behaviour and fitness to practise. 2021. Available from: https://www.gmc-uk.org/education/standards-guidance-and-curricula/guidance/student-professionalism-and-ftp/professional-behaviour-and-fitness-to-practise

8. Shrewsbury D, Mohanna K. Professionalism: Innate, caught or taught? Educ Prim Care. 2010; 21(3):199–202.

9. Kane S, Calnan M. Erosion of trust in the medical profession in India: Time for doctors to act. Int J Health Policy Manag. 2017;6(1):5–8.

10. NHS Leadership Academy. Courageous conversations. 2021. Available from: https://people.nhs.uk/guides/courageous-conversations (Accessed 27 August 21).

13

The formal, informal, and hidden curricula

Hilary Neve and Richard Nduwayezu

SUMMARY OF KEY LEARNING POINTS

■ The hidden curriculum describes the messages transmitted to learners by the culture, values, and structure of healthcare organisations and the formal curriculum.

■ The informal curriculum describes the unintended learning that usually occurs through observing and listening to role models in their daily work.

■ Learning from the informal and hidden curricula is unplanned and can have a powerful impact on learners and their professional development.

■ There are many ways of mitigating the negative effects of the informal and hidden curricula.

■ Family practice can be a very effective place to harness the positive potential of the informal and hidden curricula.

The formal curriculum

When designing an educational programme, we usually focus on the formal, or official, curriculum. The formal curriculum defines what we intend students to learn, and how we intend them to do this.[1] This involves discussing and agreeing upon the following:

■ *The purpose of the course:* What are the overall aims and learning outcomes for this course? What do we want students to know, understand, or be able to do once they have completed it?

■ *The content of the course:* What specific knowledge, skills, and attitudes do students need to learn in order to meet these learning outcomes?

■ *Learning activities:* What approaches would best help students meet each learning outcome (e.g. problem-based learning, lectures, practical skills sessions, clinical experience)?

DOI: 10.1201/9781003325734-15

- *The structure and organisation of content:* What is the best stage and order to introduce this learning and how much time is needed? How can activities build on students' previous learning?

- *Teachers and learning facilitators:* Who can best support this learning (e.g. doctors, pharmacists, nurses, patients)?

- *Assessment:* What will be assessed, what is the best approach (e.g. practical skills assessment, reflective essays, multiple choice questions), and how can we ensure students receive useful feedback?

The informal and hidden curricula

The hidden and informal curricula run in parallel with, but outside of, the planned formal curriculum[2] and describe the learning that occurs during an education course or programme which is not planned or intended (Figure 13.1). The hidden nature of these curricula means we are often not aware of their existence, or what students are learning from them. Research shows that informal and hidden learning can have a major, often negative, impact on students and their professional development.[3] However, students

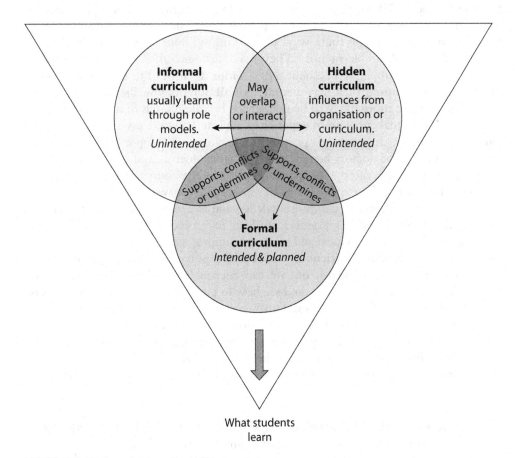

FIGURE 13.1 The formal, informal and hidden curricula.

themselves may not realise this is occurring. Learning from the informal and hidden curricula can conflict with, or undermine, the planned elements of the formal curriculum, described above. The next section explores these issues in more detail.

> Learning from the informal and hidden curricula can conflict with, undermine, or support, the planned elements of the formal curriculum.

The informal curriculum

The informal curriculum describes the spontaneous, unplanned, and unintended learning that occurs when students observe and listen to clinicians and teachers as they interact with patients, families, and colleagues, demonstrate clinical and communication skills, and explain their thinking processes. Such role modelling can help students learn to adapt to their new clinical environment and develop professionally.[4] These experiences also shape students' "basic assumptions about what are 'acceptable' and 'unacceptable' medical practices".[5]

These unplanned experiences can, however, have unforeseen and often unhelpful consequences. When students see a doctor breach confidentiality, be rude to a junior staff member, or fail to involve a patient in decisions about their care, they may unconsciously imitate these ways of working without critically reflecting on whether they are desirable or not.[4] They may also generalise out from a specific experience. For example, if a student sees a senior doctor fail to show compassion when a patient is upset, they may assume that all doctors lose their empathy over time.[6] Learners are more likely to be influenced by role models of higher status.[3]

Common informal curriculum experiences reported by students include discrimination, dishonesty, hierarchical practice, derogatory or inappropriate humour, unethical practice, or doctors being critical of other doctors and health professionals.[3,7,8] Role models are often just repeating habitual behaviours rather than purposefully communicating these messages.[9] They are usually unaware of the conflict they can create between learners' taught knowledge and the real-world clinical environment.[10] As a result of such experiences, students may become less ethical, idealistic, and empathic[2,7] and more cynical and tolerant of unprofessional behaviours.[11]

However, the informal curriculum can also be positive.[6,12] Observing role models who demonstrate high standards of care can deepen learners' understanding, help them refine and extend their skills, and see how to put learning from the formal curriculum into practice. Role models in family practice settings can play a vital role in developing students' understanding of professionalism,[13,14] teamworking, and patient-centred[15,16] holistic care.[13] Such experiences can help counteract any negative messages students have absorbed previously from other settings. Table 13.1 shows how learning from informal curriculum experiences may be positive, negative, and unpredictable.

> Role models in family practice settings can play a vital role in developing students' understanding of professionalism and holistic, patient-centred care.

TABLE 13.1 Examples of the informal curriculum in family practice

Example	What unintended or unforeseen learning may students take from this?
Observing a doctor dismiss a nurse's opinion, even though the nurse has specific, relevant expertise	• That nurses' opinions should not be valued. The students themselves may become dismissive of nurses' views and expertise • While the formal curriculum teaches us the importance of the multidisciplinary team, it does not seem valued in the real world • Students may feel upset or confused by the conflict between their formal curriculum and their real-world experience
Students see a doctor exhibit closed body language when talking to a patient who presents late in their illness and then criticise the patient for the severity of their symptoms	• Students may imitate these assumptions and behaviour when talking to patients in the future, failing to explore possible reasons for late attendance • They may be upset and decide never to talk to patients like this themselves • They may conclude that doctors become less patient-centred and empathic over time
Students hear positive messages from hospital consultants about the importance of family medicine, including examples of excellent practice	• Family practitioners play a valuable role in patients' health and are valued by consultants • This can help counteract negative stereotypes and increase students' interest in a family practice career
Student comes to know a patient well whilst on family practice placement who then dies suddenly. The supervising doctor makes time to discuss ways of managing emotions and stress	• Getting to know patients well is an advantage of family practice, that also has risks • It is OK for doctors, new and experienced, to feel emotional when bad things happen to patients. It is important to talk about and have strategies to help with this • Students may choose future jobs where the team is supportive

The hidden curriculum

The hidden curriculum is different to the informal curriculum, although there is some overlap. It describes the messages communicated to learners through the culture, structure, and perceived values of an organisation (such as a medical school, family practice, or health centre) or formal curriculum.[2] As with the informal curriculum, these messages can have a negative or positive effect on students.

Students' experiences of hierarchy, seeing how decisions are made and by whom, how they see staff being treated, and whether organisations have processes to reduce discrimination and improve quality, will all influence students' views on leadership and management, healthcare delivery, and may determine their career choices.[8] Students will also, subconsciously, be influenced by how the formal curriculum is designed; their ideas about what is important in medicine will be shaped by what is taught, what is not taught, how much time is allocated for different topics, and what is, or is not, assessed. Their views on different professions may be influenced by who is invited to teach (consultants, family doctors, or other health professionals) and their views on different population groups by how they are represented in teaching materials.[17]

Students often struggle emotionally when they witness behaviours which conflict with what they have been taught.

As with the informal curriculum, the hidden curriculum can be a force for good. Students' experiences in family practice, particularly if longitudinal, can be hugely influential. Seeing how family practices facilitate effective teamwork, organise and adapt systems to meet the needs of disadvantaged groups, or learn together in practice can shape students' understanding of professionalism and effective healthcare delivery. They may also challenge misconceptions about a career in family practice. Table 13.2 demonstrates how learning from hidden curriculum experiences may be positive or negative.

Students' experiences of the hidden curriculum in family practice can have a huge positive influence and may help challenge career stereotypes.

TABLE 13.2 Examples of the hidden curriculum in family practice

Example	What unintended or unforeseen learning may students take from this?
FM placements last a week and learning is not assessed. Surgical placements are four weeks long and have a formal assessment	• Learning about surgery and anatomy is more important than learning about family practice • They may be reluctant to pursue a career that does not seem valued by their school
Educational case studies perpetuate stereotypes, e.g. heart disease cases are always men, or cases involving depression or domestic violence are always women	• Some health issues only affect certain demographic groups, e.g. women do not have cardiovascular disease and/or men do not experience depression or domestic violence • They may feel frustrated that their family or friends' demographic is not fairly represented
Patients are invited to a workshop to share their varied personal stories of managing diabetes. When they share difficult experiences, patients begin to support each other	• Different patients have different experiences of the same illness and want different things from their care • Patients can play an important role supporting each other • Students may ask to help set up a patient support group
During their family practice placement, students see the whole team have a daily timetabled coffee break where they discuss patients, share difficulties, and support each other	• Teamwork and mutual support is important, but you have to make time to foster it • You will not know all the answers and others can help and offer important new perspectives

When designing a curriculum, it is important to consider how to minimise negative hidden and informal curriculum messages and maximise positive messages.

Addressing the informal and hidden curricula

There are many things family practice educators do about the hidden and informal curricula:

1. When planning a curriculum, discuss the values you are aiming to communicate and how your curriculum can reflect these. What negative messages might your curriculum communicate to students? How could you minimise these?

2. Ensure your educator team understands the aims and underpinning values of the curriculum, and how you define professionalism (Chapter 12). This will help role models to communicate informal messages which support, rather than conflict with, the formal curriculum

3. Tell your team about the informal curriculum, the potential risks, and the benefits of role modelling (Chapter 16).[4] Explain that students will often take a casual throw-away remark or jokey comment seriously.[3] Suggest they all reflect on any negative messages they may have communicated to learners and consider how to be more effective role models in the future.

4. Explain that being a positive role model does not mean being perfect! Encourage educators to be honest with students when things do not go well and to demonstrate how they reflect on, and learn from, this. Suggest they talk about difficult issues they have faced in FM, such as medical error, stress, conflicting demands, and home–work balance, and how they have learnt to address these. These can be powerful learning experiences for students.

5. Tell students that the hidden and informal curricula exist and explain how these can impact on their learning and development. This can be eye-opening for students.[6] Encourage students to look out for positive and negative experiences of the informal or hidden curriculum and reflect critically on these and their potential impact in writing, or with peers. This can help raise awareness and mitigate negative effects.[6,14]

6. Ensure there are clear processes for students to report any unprofessional behaviour they experience and that these are acted upon. Students often struggle emotionally when they witness behaviours which conflict with what they have been taught, but when faculty appear to tolerate these, this can lead to strong feelings of powerlessness and hopelessness in students.[17]

Learning about the existence of the hidden and informal curricula can be eye-opening for students and educators.

Conclusion

The hidden and formal curricula can have a major impact on a learner's professional development. While this chapter has focused on undergraduates, similar issues affect learners across the health professions at all stages of their career. It is important that teachers and curriculum designers know about these curricula in order to minimise any negative messages and harness the benefits. However, the concepts of the hidden and informal curricula can be hard for teachers and students to grasp; they may struggle particularly with the unconscious and hidden nature of these messages and how they have unintended and unpredictable effects. Yet understanding these concepts can be empowering for both students and educators.

References

1. Gill D. Course design. In: Cantillon P, Wood DF, Yardley S. (eds.), ABC of learning and teaching in medicine. 3rd ed. Oxford: John Wiley & Sons; 2017. pp. 15–18.
2. Doja A, Bould MD, Clarkin C, Eady K, Sutherland S, Writer H. The hidden and informal curriculum across the continuum of training: A cross-sectional qualitative study. Med Educ. 2016;38(4):410–18.
3. Mahood SC. Medical education: Beware the hidden curriculum. Can Fam Physician. 2011;57(9):983–85.
4. Benbassat J. Role modelling in medical education: The importance of a reflective imitation. Acad Med. 2014;89(4):550–54.
5. Haidet P, Stein HF. The role of the student–teacher relationship in the formation of physicians. J Gen Intern Med. 2006;21(1):16–20.
6. Neve H, Collett T. Empowering students with the hidden curriculum. Clin Teach. 2018;15(6):494–99.
7. Yahyavi ST, Hoobehfekr S, Tabatabaee M. Exploring the hidden curriculum of professionalism and medical ethics in a psychiatry emergency department. Asian J Psychiatr. 2021;66:102885.
8. Wass V, Gregory S, Petty-Saphon K. By choice—not by chance: Supporting medical students towards future careers in general practice. London: Health Education England and the Medical Schools Council; 2016.
9. Merton RK. The unanticipated consequences of purposive social action. Am Sociol Rev. 1936;1(6):894–904.
10. Berger P, Luckmann T. The social construction of reality. New York: Anchor Books; 1967.
11. Peng J, Clarkin C, Doja A. Uncovering cynicism in medical training: A qualitative analysis of medical online discussion forums. BMJ Open. 2018;8(10):e022883.
12. Almairi SO, Sajid MR, Azouz R, Mohamed RR, Almairi M, Fadul T. Students' and faculty perspectives toward the role and value of the hidden curriculum in undergraduate medical education: A qualitative study from Saudi Arabia. Med Sci Educ. 2021;31(2):753–64.
13. Roberts C, Daly M, Kumar K, Perkins D, Richards D, Garne D. A longitudinal integrated placement and medical students' intentions to practise rurally. Med Educ. 2012;46(2):179–91.
14. Karnieli-Miller O, Vu TR, Frankel RM, Holtman MC, Clyman SG, Hui SL, Inui TS. Which experiences in the hidden curriculum teach students about professionalism? Acad Med. 2011;86(3):369–77.
15. Pagatpatan Jr CP, Valdezco JA, Lauron JD. Teaching the affective domain in community-based medical education: A scoping review. Med Teach. 2020;42(5):507–14.
16. White CB, Kumagai AK, Ross PT, Fantone JC. A qualitative exploration of how the conflict between the formal and informal curriculum influences student values and behaviours. Acad Med. 2009;84(5):597–603.
17. Marcelin JR, Siraj DS, Victor R, Kotadia S, Maldonado YA. The impact of unconscious bias in healthcare: How to recognize and mitigate it. J Infect Dis. 2019;220(Suppl. 2):S62–S73.

Integrating FM into the curriculum

How to achieve this

Do not confine children to your own learning for they were born in another time.

Hebrew proverb

14

Selecting for medical school entry
Nature or nurture?

Sandra Nicholson and Tim J. Wilkinson

SUMMARY OF KEY LEARNING POINTS

■ Selection into medical school is risky—for applicants who invest heavily in securing a place at medical school, for medical schools who need to choose those applicants who will graduate, and for society wishing to secure a highly competent healthcare workforce.

■ The end product, i.e. the graduate, combines what individuals bring to the programme (nature) with what is gained by undertaking the programme (nurture).

■ Involving family doctors in all stages of medical school selection helps ensure successful applicants hold appropriate values and aptitudes.

■ Whilst research into medical selection has increased, we still lack high-quality theory-driven studies.

■ Significant evidence on the utility and predictive validity of common selection tools exists to inform medical school selection policy and practice.

■ Selection processes must move towards shaping a future workforce and not just predicting success within a programme.

Introduction and background

Selection into the medical profession is often called "high stakes" because the people involved can gain or lose a great deal.[1] Stakes are high for the public as poor decisions place patients at risk by selecting applicants unable to take on demanding roles. They are high for applicants as its competitive nature requires time, energy, and money to prepare. Scrutiny of medical school selection processes is mandatory to ensure they are fit for purpose and remain so. Established selection practices have been challenged by the need to achieve effective global workforce planning, including recruitment into family medicine (FM) and creating greater diversity of the medical profession.

DOI: 10.1201/9781003325734-17

Selection processes for primary care training are high stakes too. The attributes needed can relate more to a practitioner's motivations and personality than those learnt in medical school. Family doctors add value to medical school selection processes by informing the desired characteristics of graduating cohorts of doctors to ensure successful applicants have the necessary experiences and motivations for generalist care.

> Selection into medical school remains high stakes for applicants, medical schools, patients, and society.

This chapter outlines current challenges in medical school selection as shared by most countries, provides an update on selection practices, discusses what values-based selection means, and explores how these issues may impact upon FM recruitment. The principles also apply to selection into postgraduate medical training.

Current challenges to medical school selection

Lack of high-quality research

The evidence base for selection has advanced significantly since the 2018 consensus statement drawn up by Patterson et al.[2] Some of its recommendations remain elusive. Box 14.1 summarises issues relevant to selection into FM.

There is clear evidence that prior academic attainment is a strong predictor of subsequent performance within a programme and in postgraduate examinations. This should not be the only selection criterion.[3] Some selection tools are known to be unreliable, e.g. personal statements and references, yet these remain commonly used by some. Patterson et al. highlight the lack of utilisable research to inform selection policies, particularly those related to health outcomes.[4,5]

BOX 14.1 SUMMARY OF SELECTED RECOMMENDATIONS FROM 2018 CONSENSUS STATEMENT THAT HIGHLIGHT ISSUES RELEVANT TO SELECTION FOR FM[2]

1. Identify behaviours needed for success as a healthcare practitioner.
2. Develop ways to evaluate selection methodologies that take differences in context into account and relate to health outcomes.
3. Consider the social accountability of the training programmes to support social inclusion, workforce issues, government and institutional policy, and the patient perspective.
4. Consider how taking an interdisciplinary approach may facilitate the future development of selection policy and practice by using appropriate methodologies sensitive to local contextual priorities, e.g. recruitment of future family doctors.

Lack of clear markers of success

What are the markers of success in selection? This is a fundamental question. Many have presumed that it is predictive validity, i.e. how well do selection tools predict performance within the course? However, within medicine, nearly all those selected graduate. A better quality marker might be how well selection tools result in a "fit for purpose" workforce.

> The lack of high-quality research into medical selection, and lack of clarity on what indicates an effective selection process, limit selection and workforce planning policy development.

Fairness, diversity, and representation

Many selection processes, however well intended, inadvertently exclude people from under-represented groups, particularly those liable to societal inequities and lesser opportunities. Sometimes selection processes assess specific skills that could subsequently be learnt during the programme or ones which unrepresented groups have had insufficient opportunities to develop, e.g. more traditional academic skills. In many countries, the level of school leavers' exam achievement is more reflective of their socio-economic status than their ability. To avoid exclusion of under-represented groups, attention to these inadvertent adverse consequences is required. Instead of ranking on attribute performance to select the "best" performers, stating a threshold to be achieved is potentially fairer. In other words, what is good enough to be able to successfully complete the programme?

> Excluding from under-represented groups risks generating a workforce which fails to mirror the population it serves.

Ensuring best selection practice: What criteria should be used?

"When you're a hammer, everything looks like a nail" describes a traditional approach to selection. It is tempting to select a tool and then decide how best to use it. This approach is misguided. It is important to step back and first ask: (i) "What is the purpose of the selection process?" (ii) What is being looked for? (iii) Should we use selection criteria for "what is needed to practise" or for "what is needed to complete the programme"? There can be a tendency to select on the end product, e.g. the qualities of "the good health professional". This ignores the fact that the end product combines what is gained by undertaking the programme (nurture) with what individuals bring to the programme (nature). We propose it makes more sense to select on aspects that cannot be learnt on the programme.

$$\underset{\text{practice (end-product)}}{\text{What is needed in}} - \underset{\text{programme (nurture)}}{\text{What is learnt in the}} = \underset{\text{selection (nature)}}{\text{What is needed in}}$$

Intended learning outcomes document what is learnt in the programme. Sometimes, but not always, what is needed in practice is described by the programme goals but is oftentimes broader than this and poses a question partly for society to answer.

Here are some suggested outcomes that a selection process could assess:

1. Aptitude to undertake the programme
2. Mirror on society—the health practitioner profile should reflect the values and demographics of the society they will serve
3. Generic skills, e.g. communication, empathy, and honesty
4. Specific skills, e.g. content knowledge, consultation skills, procedural skills
5. Aptitude for ongoing learning

Training programmes nurture by ensuring specific skills are met and by building on the required generic skills. Values and learning aptitudes can be influenced positively or negatively by the curriculum but also reflect learner motivation. However, a training programme cannot change demographics or teach aptitudes. A selection process should therefore focus on the "nature components", i.e. values, demographics, and aptitudes, to undertake the programme. It may highlight some generic skills and motivation but need not select on those skills that can be taught. Traditionally, merit has been equated with academic success. Widening the approach to selection, as we suggest, requires active consideration of what else constitutes merit.[6]

It is important to define what values, demographics, and aptitudes are being looked for in applicants and not the skills which can be learnt on the programme.

Ensuring best selection practice: How should we assess?

As for any complex area, medical school selection requires a mix of tools, blueprinted to the attributes being looked for,[7] while ensuring the process is feasible and acceptable. Most selection strategies employ an initial screening to cope with high applicant numbers, use more criteria than academic achievement alone, and include an opportunity to meet candidates. A systematic review by Patterson et al. identifies outcomes of research into the effectiveness, strengths and weaknesses, and psychometrics (including reliability and validity) of selection methods.[8] Table 14.1 summarises the main available tools.

TABLE 14.1 Common tools used for selection into medical school

Tool	Description	Advantages	Disadvantages
Early screening			
Academic grades	Aggregate of assessment results from a course	Readily available; often predict course performance	Restrict measurable attributes; inequitable for learners from disadvantaged backgrounds; limited utility
Personal statement	Applicants outline their qualities	Easy implementation; highly acceptable	Problems with authenticating who wrote the statement. Poor predictive validity
Shortlisting for interview			
Aptitude tests	Commercial psychometric tests; often online	Facilitate discrimination Easy to use	Variability across tests; mixed evidence on predictive validity; debate on fairness if widening participation the aim
Written personality tests	Assess personality traits less prone to change	May be useful to "rule out" rather than "rule in"	Heterogeneous in quality and evidence; maybe susceptible to coaching, limited evidence of outcomes, and utility
Later: Face-to-face assessment (online or virtual)			
Interview	Between applicant and one or more selectors	Assesses attributes in depth (e.g. communication)	If unstructured, unreliable and prone to bias. Standardised questions and interviewer training can improve reliability
Multiple mini-interview (MMI)	OSCE format of multiple stations and assessors	Wider in-depth assessment of attributes	Increased reliability as more cases and assessors used. Resource-intensive. Issues concerning construct validity
References	Written statement attesting candidate's suitability	May be useful to "rule out" rather than "rule in"	Variable in quality. Low validity and reliability
Situational judgement tests	Test attributes mapped to organisational values	Improved validity Deliverable online	Relatively costly to design
Selection centre: Small group activity	Applicant does tasks aligned to the actual job	High validity	Expensive, unfeasible for large numbers of applicants
Lottery	Random selection. Can be after academic screening	Superficial fairness. Low costs	Candidates dislike process

Many methods are discussed in Chapters 27 and 29 on Assessment. Readers may be less familiar with multi-mini interviews (MMIs) and situational judgement tests (SJTs), both in common use.

MMIs use multiple stations through which candidates rotate, similar to the structure of an Objective Structured Clinical Examination (OSCE). At each station, they may be interviewed, presented with a scenario, or asked to undertake a task. The stations assess a balance of the desired attributes. Their advantage, as for OSCEs, is gaining multiple samples of a candidate's performance and multiple examiner judgements. Sampling from a range of attributes increases validity while multiple samples of each applicant increase reliability. MMIs have increased predictive validity over other assessment tools.[9,10]

SJTs are traditionally presented in multiple choice format. The questions are posed as professional dilemmas a candidate might face in their work and where more than one answer could be appropriate. Candidates' answers can be weighted rather than simply marked right or wrong. The scenarios are usually appropriate to contexts a candidate might encounter, i.e. those relevant to a school leaver rather than medicine. SJTs attempt to assess professional judgement. There is increasing evidence that they achieve this.[11] It is also possible that SJTs could be suitably designed to increase selection for FM.

Published evidence shows that MMIs, SJTs, academic records, and aptitude tests are more valid and reliable selection tools than traditional interviews, references, and personal statements.

Ensuring best selection practice for FM values-based recruitment (VBR)

As we broaden selection criteria beyond the traditional academic achievement, are we neglecting to emphasise specific personal qualities required for a career in FM? This highlights the importance of including a values-based recruitment (VBR) approach into healthcare selection.[1] Best practice articulates that a thorough job analysis should be completed to identify which attributes and, hence which selection tools, should be used. Many would argue that there is a commonality of competency, trainability, and aptitude across all medical specialties.[12]

Yet, internationally, FM has evolved significantly adapting to global health needs, e.g. obesity, ageing, and multimorbidity, maternal and child morbidity, and conditions exacerbated by poor sanitation and nutrition. Understanding the impact of public health on patients' needs is just as necessary as discussing lifestyle choices. Globally, the COVID-19 pandemic has changed FM forever. The use of telecommunications and managing risk without directly examining patients requires a different skill set.

To ensure we select for the future workforce, now is the time for a range of practitioners, including family doctors, to reset selection criteria, agree on assessment tools to use, and ensure all stakeholders engage in the process. A word of warning, this selection approach cannot guarantee we specifically select for FM. Most students decide their career choices after graduation or change their minds whilst studying, but it does emphasise the values and aptitudes required to succeed as a family doctor.[13,14]

Healthcare delivery is changing, defining the values underpinning future FM practice is important when selecting medical students.

A CASE STUDY ON VALUES-BASED RECRUITMENT IN NEW ZEALAND

Indigenous people (Māori) are under-represented within the New Zealand medical workforce. Yet, if the health workforce represents the population, Māori health outcomes are known to be better. Māori students have been under-represented in medical school. This related to lower expectations set at secondary school and to selection processes. To address this, a multipronged approach was taken. Outreach programmes to schools were implemented to inform future students of health professional career options and their requirements. The selection processes were altered; for some attributes, a threshold only was needed, and ranking was made on other attributes. Despite some resistance by traditionally privileged groups and claims of unfairness, addressing historical inequities is not only legal, but desirable. Support was then offered, where needed, within medical school. The medical degree graduation rates for Māori are no different from other groups. The Māori proportion in medical schools is now greater than the population levels, although the health workforce inequities will take longer to correct.[6,15]

Selection processes need to ensure suitable people are targeted well before the selection process and supported once they enter a programme.

Conclusion and areas for future research

There is good evidence on the effectiveness of some selection tools in predicting success within a course. More work is needed to focus selection on the attributes to select for, not just the tools, and on shaping a workforce that suits societal needs.

Five tips for global recruitment

1. Gain consensus on the attributes to select for.

2. Select innate attributes which cannot be learnt within the training programme.

3. Consider societal needs on the makeup of a suitable workforce.

4. Use selection tools that have a good evidence base, including candidate acceptability, utility, validity, reliability, and cost-effectiveness.

5. Utilise a variety of selection modalities to assess the values required for FM.

References

1. Patterson F, Zibarras I (eds.). Selection and recruitment in the healthcare professions: Research, theory and practice. Cham: Palgrave Macmillan; 2018.

2. Patterson F, Roberts C, Hanson MD, Hampe W, Eva K, Ponnamperuma G, Magzoub M, Tekian A, Cleland J. Ottawa consensus statement: Selection and recruitment to the healthcare professions. Med Teach. 2018;40(11):1091–101. doi: 10.1080/0142159X.2018.1498589

3. McManus I, Woolf K, Dacre J et al. The academic backbone: Longitudinal continuities in educational achievement from secondary school and medical school to MRCP(UK) and the specialist register in UK medical students and doctors. BMC Med. 2013;11:242. doi: 10.1186/1741-7015-11-242

4. Patterson F, Cleland J, Cousans F. Selection methods in healthcare professions: Where are we now and where next? Adv Health Sci Educ. 2017;22(2):229–42. doi: 10.1007/s10459-017-9752-7

5. Gorman D. Matching the production of doctors with national needs. Med Educ. 2018;152:103–13.

6. Crampton P, Baxter J, Bristowe Z. Selection of Māori students into medicine: Re-imagining merit. Exploring some of the sociological reasons that might explain the exclusion of Māori from the medical workforce. N Z Med J. 2021;134(1543):59.

7. Wilkinson TM, Wilkinson TJ. Selection into medical school: From tools to domains. BMC Med Educ. 2016;16(1):1–6.

8. Patterson F, Knight A, Dowell J, Nicholson S, Cousans F, Cleland J. How effective are selection methods in medical education? A systematic review. Med Educ. 2016;50(1):36–60.

9. Eva KW, Rosenfeld J, Reiter HI, Norman GR. An admissions OSCE: The multiple mini-interview. Med Educ. 2004;38(3):314–26.

10. Eva KW, Reiter HI, Trinh K, Wasi P, Rosenfeld J, Norman GR. Predictive validity of the multiple mini-interview for selecting medical trainees. Med Educ. 2009;43(8):767–75.

11. Patterson F, Zibarras L, Ashworth V. Situational judgement tests in medical education and training: Research, theory and practice: AMEE Guide No. 100.Med Teach. 2016;38(1):3–17. doi:10.3109/0142159X.2015.1072619.

12. Patterson F, Tavabie A, Denney M, et al. A new competency model for general practice; Implications for selection, training, and careers. Br J Gen Pract. 2013;63(610):e331–8.

13. Cleland JA, Johnston PW, Anthony M, Khan N, Scott NW. A survey of factors influencing career preference in new-entrant and exiting medical students from four UK medical schools. BMC Med Educ. 2014;14:151.

14. Pfarrwaller E, Voirol L, Piumatti G, Karemera M, Sommer J, Gerbase MW, Guerrier S, Baroffio A. Students' intentions to practice primary care are associated with their motives to become doctors: A longitudinal study. BMC Med Educ. 2022;22(1):30.

15. Crampton P, Weaver N, Howard A. Holding a mirror to society? The sociodemographic characteristics of the University of Otago's health professional students. N Z Med J. 2012;125(1361):12–28.

15

Early exposure to family medicine

Victor Loh and Innocent Besigye

SUMMARY OF KEY LEARNING POINTS

- Exposure to primary care and family medicine (FM) educators early in medical school (traditionally in the "preclinical years") is important.
- FM educators role model holistic, relationship-based, person-centred community care by integrating psychosocial aspects of health with biomedical aspects of disease.
- Early exposure to FM in undergraduate training redresses healthcare fragmentation from an overemphasis on super-specialisation and biomedical aspects of disease.
- Authentic patient contact in primary care socialises learners to the community context and reinforces the importance of humanistic values and good communication in medical professional identity formation.
- Learning in the community, where the bulk of medicine is practised, supports deeper situational learning, enabling and motivating learners to link and apply their basic sciences to the clinical context in which they will practise.
- Early FM exposure is an important strategy for increasing vocational uptake in FM.

Introduction

The traditional biomedical model

In 1910, Abraham Flexner produced a report that transformed medical education first in America and then worldwide.[1] Ever since then, the disease–based biomedical model has taken precedence in medical schools globally. While endorsement of the scientific basis of medicine initially benefitted medical training and practice, we now experience, to varying extents, the unintended effects of Flexner's report. We face a hyperemphasis on the *Science of Medicine* to the detriment of the *Art of Medicine* in medical training and clinical practice. This has challenged educators preparing future doctors

DOI: 10.1201/9781003325734-18

for a more value-based healthcare which places patients and population needs at the centre of clinical care and focuses more on well-being and the social determinants of health alongside the need to apply disease-based scientific evidence to the increasing complexity of multimorbidity and polypharmacy.

> Modern health delivery places the patient at the centre of care rather than the disease. Medical education must adapt to rebalance the Art with the Science of medicine.

We see echoes of this in the way medical school curricula are typically sequenced, with a strong biomedical emphasis in the preclinical years, followed by hospital specialist and super-specialist clinical postings in the later clinical years. This reflects healthcare systems worldwide which are often organised around acute care hospitals with priority and funding given to hospital-specialist departments. The role of the community primary care specialist is often an afterthought. As a result, medical care becomes fragmented, depersonalised, episodic, and hospital-based, with a weak doctor–patient relationship.

The evolving ecology of medical care has consistently shown, where healthcare systems are organised around strong primary care, that there is usually little reason for hospital referral or admission for persons in the community.[2] Unfortunately, medical training is often largely secondary or tertiary care-based with inpatient placements within specialised hospitals. Students are thus trained mainly for the hospital setting. Ironically, they then graduate lacking the generalist expertise and attributes necessary for whole-person care in the community where the bulk of healthcare professionals will eventually work.

While over the years, since the 1960s, progress has been made to redress this with, for example, the establishment of boards of family practice in the United States and of FM departments in various universities, the fragmentation persists. In 2010, a Lancet Commission[3] confirmed that health professional training remained fragmented and mainly hospital based. It argued strongly that to produce fit-for purpose graduates for the 21st century, healthcare education must change.

> To produce healthcare professionals for the 21st century, a move towards increased community FM-based placements where generalist skills can be learnt is essential.

Early family medicine exposure

We define early exposure to FM as any curricular interaction with FM educators in the "preclinical years" which would typically mean the first two or three years of most international programmes or equivalent.[4,5]

Early exposure can take various forms: *Clinical placements*, through regular visits to primary care across the academic year and/or discrete FM blocks, meet students' desire to interact early in the curriculum with patients, and motivate learning as they can apply a real-world context to classroom medical science lessons.[4–6] Alternatives include *longitudinal integrated clerkships* (Chapter 17) or *student projects in the community*, e.g. health screening projects, sometimes as student-selected activities. Students experience family physicians role modelling holistic care of patients and families in their homes and communities. In general, the greater the frequency and dosage of positive early year experiences in the real-world primary care setting, the greater the effect on FM as a subsequent vocational choice.[7]

Where finding placements is an issue, an alternative is to *bring family physician educators into campus* to facilitate learning. FM faculty can co-design and/or co-teach with medical science colleagues and bring medical science learning to life by drawing on experiences and case discussions of community patient care. Through observation of tutors role modelling holistic community care and/or hearing their stories, students may reflect on and appreciate FM values and the crucial role family physicians play in the community delivering primary healthcare to persons and families.

> FM educators from early in the medical school curriculum act as powerful role models of the generalist person-centred care they deliver in the community.

Socialisation of medical students

Placing students in primary care socialises them to the clinical and societal context of where and how FM work occurs. It is important to design learning outcomes which actively involve students in the life and functions of the clinic. For instance, lesson plans could entail learner interactions with walk-in patients from the community, who speak with unfamiliar dialects, or local forms of expression. It is important that students listen to and value the patient's narrative in the context of their family and psychosocial circumstances. This may open the student's eyes to cultures and socio-economic conditions with which they are unfamiliar (Chapter 12). They can learn to register, interview, and report to the FM tutor on the patient's story and reason for attending.

Working alongside FM tutors and the healthcare team situates medical training in the community context where many will eventually practice. Entrusting students with stage-appropriate tasks in patient care, while working alongside family physicians, strengthens learner's confidence in interactions with patients,[6,8] reduces learner's stress during transitions to clinical clerkships,[4,9,10] and opens opportunities for mentorship.[11] Importantly, it strengthens medical professional identity formation and seeds FM as a viable vocational choice.[11,12]

Contextualisation of classroom learning

Early clinical placements build on the sociocultural theory of situational learning. They enable students to contextualise classroom learning in the real-world setting which enhances deeper more long-term recall of learning. For example, taking a history of a presenting complaint and eliciting clinical signs from a real patient gives life to lectures in anatomy and physiology among other basic science subjects. Listening to parental concerns around their child's health risk behaviour gives life to lessons on the social and affective factors that influence health. First-hand observations of the doctor–patient relationship gives life to discussions on ethics and professionalism. In addition, the primary care setting is excellent for learning clinical skills.[13]

Enabling students to connect knowledge from the classroom with real-life clinical experience results in deeper situational learning.

Thus, early FM exposure embeds scientific learning more deeply,[6] provides respite from the classroom,[10] and reinforces and motivates learning[4,5,8] by connecting classroom lessons with the very real health problems of patients who access healthcare by walking into family practices right at the doorstep of the community where they live and work.

Humanisation of medical care

Opportunities to interact with patients and their families in their communities humanise medical training and care (Chapter 7). Meeting actual patients early in medical school reminds students of the reasons they joined the vocation. It anchors the fundamental understanding that medical training is about caring for the *patient as a person with a family*, a *sociocultural context*, and a *personal narrative* who is experiencing illness. It redresses the biomedical hyper-emphasis on disease(s) or body parts as the focus of curriculum planning.

Observation of the doctor–patient relationship, and of holistic care in practice, allows the recognition of how the social, behavioural, and ethical sciences are relevant to medical training. It demonstrates how health systems succeed or fail in providing access to care.[6] Students learn to empathise with others and to reflect on their own inadequacies and uncertainties in relating meaningfully with patients and their complexities.[14]

Box 15.1 summarises the roles of early FM clinical exposure as an educational intervention.

Educators and patients have in turn found engaging with students early in their studies motivating and rewarding. Early clinical experiences remind us all that the *art* of medicine matters; that understanding the psychosocial aspects of care is crucial. It reaffirms for learners the meaning and purpose of medical training.[15]

Interacting and empathising with patients and observing FM role models early in their career helps students build their professional identity.

While clearly a valuable educational intervention, we recognise the challenges involved in delivering early FM clinical placements. We share some tips on how these may be implemented and encourage innovation to optimise opportunities whatever the primary care and community structures in your setting.

BOX 15.1 THE ROLE OF EARLY FM CLINICAL EXPOSURE AS AN EDUCATIONAL INTERVENTION

Early FM clinical exposure

Socialises medical students to the clinical workplace in the community, provides confidence in transitions to the clinical environment, and strengthens medical professional identity formation.

Contextualises classroom learning of the basic sciences, social determinants of health, ethical and professional practice, and clinical skills training to the real-world setting beyond the hospital; motivates student learning.

Humanises medical training and practice. Observation of FM attributes-in-action reminds learners that the goal of medical training is the holistic care of *persons*.

Implementing early FM exposure in medical school

1. Involve FM educators early in the curriculum:

Start with involving FM educators as early as possible in the curriculum. Some medical schools start community placements in week 1. Others with campus medical science sessions as a base have placements across the year or provide opportunities for FM faculty to teach with medical scientists using community case studies to illustrate learning points. Keep in mind the value of providing a platform for students to interact with FM educators, and for positive FM role models to be introduced as early as possible in the curriculum.

2. Insert placements in FM and the community:

Insert regular FM clinical placements as soon, and as frequently, as possible, across the early years. Link these longitudinally for frequent exposure to the FM setting to occur. Longitudinal integrated clerkships (Chapter 17) are an effective strategy for early exposure to the social and clinical contexts of FM. Maximise different placement opportunities wherever you can.

3. Link lesson plans to classroom sessions:

Integrate ongoing medical science classroom curricula with lesson plans in the clinical setting. For example, during a cardiovascular system block, task students to ask about cardiovascular complaints, or instruct students to take the blood pressure of patients in the waiting room. Plan for learning to spiral to the clinical years (Chapter 11). Work with medical scientists in planning a curriculum that integrates with the medical sciences.

4. Emphasise the Principles of FM:

Introduce the principles and values of FM early in the curriculum and link these to vertical themes such as whole-person care, a life-course approach, professionalism, person-centred care, first contact care, and comprehensive, coordinated, and continuing care[16] (Chapter 11). Provide learners with the opportunity to appreciate the value of generalism; how the perspective of each patient as a person in space, time, and in a specific sociocultural context sensitises future practitioners to holistic patient care regardless of future-intended specialty.

5. Ensure adequate faculty training:

Faculty training is key. Ensure FM tutors are clear about the overall purpose of early clinical exposure, and that they link the lesson plan and intended learning outcomes in the community setting with classroom sessions. Develop a FM educator community of practice[17] to allow for mutual support and sharing of teaching ideas.

6. Set aside time for reflective practice:

Ensure learning occurs by setting time aside for reflective practice after each learning experience. The principles of FM are often appreciated only after reflecting on experiences at the clinic (Chapter 19). Reflection may be formal or informal, and may take the form of a reflective portfolio[18] where learners chart their learning in discussion with a trusted mentor (Chapter 26).

Conclusion

Early FM *clinical* exposure *socialises* medical students to the reality of medical practice *beyond the hospital, contextualises* and motivates classroom learning by bringing lessons to life *in the community,* and *humanises* medical learning and care right *in the neighbourhood.* Experiencing generalist care in the community rehabilitates the *biopsychosocial* model, promotes whole-person care, and strengthens FM as vocational choice among learners.

References

1. Duffy TP. The Flexner report—100 years later. Yale J Biol Med. 2011;84(3):269. Available from: https://www.ncbi.nlm.nih.gov/pmc/articles/PMC3178858/ (Accessed 21 December 2021).
2. Green LA, Fryer Jr GE, Yawn BP, Lanier D, Dovey SM. The ecology of medical care revisited. N Engl J Med. 2001;344(26):2021–5.
3. Frenk J, Chen L, Bhutta ZA, Cohen J, Crisp N, Evans T, Fineberg H, Garcia P, Ke Y, Kelley P, Kistnasamy B. Health professionals for a new century: Transforming education to strengthen health systems in an interdependent world. Lancet. 2010;376(9756): 1923–58. Available from: https://www.thelancet.com/journals/lancet/article/PIIS0140-6736(10)60450-3/fulltext
4. Dornan T, Littlewood S, Margolis SA, Scherpbier AJ, Spencer J, Ypinazar V. How can experience in clinical and community settings contribute to early medical education? A BEME systematic review. Med Teach. 2006;28(1):3–18. Available from: https://www.tandfonline.com/doi/abs/10.1080/01421590500410971 (Accessed 21 December 2021).
5. Yardley S, Littlewood S, Margolis SA, Scherpbier A, Spencer J, Ypinazar V, Dornan T. What has changed in the evidence for early experience? Update of a BEME systematic review. Med Teach. 2010;32(9):740–46. Available from: https://www.tandfonline.com/doi/abs/10.3109/0142159X.2010.496007 (Accessed 21 December 2021).
6. Orbell S, Abraham C. Behavioural sciences and the real world: Report of a community interview scheme for medical students. Med Educ. 1993;27(3):218–28. Available from: https://onlinelibrary.wiley.com/doi/abs/10.1111/j.1365-2923.1993.tb00260.x (Accessed 21 December 2021).

7. Shah A, Gasner A, Bracken K, Scott I, Kelly MA, Palombo A. Early generalist placements are associated with family medicine career choice: A systematic review and meta-analysis. Med Educ. 2021. Available from: https://onlinelibrary.wiley.com/doi/abs/10.1111/medu.14578 (Accessed 21 December 2021).

8. van Oppen J, Camm C, Sahota G, Taggar J, Knox R. Medical students' attitudes towards increasing early clinical exposure to primary care. Educ Prim Care. 2018;29(5). Available from: https://nottingham-repository.worktribe.com/index.php/output/942360/medical-students-attitudes-towards-increasing-early-clinical-exposure-to-primary-care (Accessed 21 December 2021).

9. Barley G, O'Brien-Gonzales A, Hughes E. What did we learn about the impact on students' clinical education? Acad Med. 2001;76(4):S68–S71. Available from: https://journals.lww.com/academicmedicine/Fulltext/2001/04001/What_Did_We_Learn_about_the_Impact_on_Students_.13.aspx (Accessed 21 December 2021).

10. Littlewood S, Ypinazar V, Margolis SA, Scherpbier A, Spencer J, Dornan T. Early practical experience and the social responsiveness of clinical education: Systematic review. Br Med J. 2005;331(7513):387–91. Available from: https://citeseerx.ist.psu.edu/viewdoc/download?doi=10.1.1.119.9979&rep=rep1&type=pdf (Accessed 21 December 2021).

11. John J, Brown ME. The impact of longitudinal integrated clerkships on patient care: A qualitative systematic review. Educ Prim Care. 2021:1–1. Available from: https://www.tandfonline.com/doi/abs/10.1080/14739879.2021.1980438 (Accessed 21 December 2021).

12. O'Doherty D, Culhane A, O'Doherty J, Harney S, Glynn L, McKeague H, Kelly D. Medical students and clinical placements: A qualitative study of the continuum of professional identity formation. Educ Prim Care. 2021:1–9. Available from: https://www.tandfonline.com/doi/full/10.1080/14739879.2021.1879684 (Accessed 21 December 2021).

13. Park S, Khan NF, Hampshire M, Knox R, Malpass A, Thomas J, Anagnostelis B, Newman M, Bower P, Rosenthal J, Murray E. A BEME systematic review of UK undergraduate medical education in the general practice setting: BEME Guide no. 32. Med Teach. 2015;37(7):611–30. Available from: https://www.tandfonline.com/doi/abs/10.3109/0142159X.2015.1032918 (Accessed 21 December 2021).

14. Kent GG. Medical students' reactions to a nursing attachment scheme. Med Educ. 1991;25(1):23–31. Available from: https://onlinelibrary.wiley.com/doi/abs/10.1111/j.1365-2923.1991.tb00022.x (Accessed 21 December 2021).

15. Freeman J, Cash C, Yonke A, Roe B, Foley R. A longitudinal primary care program in an urban public medical school: Three years of experience. Acad Med J Assoc Am Med Coll. 1995;70(1 Suppl.):S64–S8. Available from: https://europepmc.org/article/med/7826460 (Accessed 21 December 2021).

16. Allen J, Gay B, Crebolder H, Heyrman J, Svab I, Ram P, Evans P. The European definition of general practice/family medicine. WONCA Europe. 2011. Available from: https://www.globalfamilydoctor.com/site/DefaultSite/filesystem/documents/regionDocs/European%20Definition%20of%20general%20practice%203rd%20ed%202011.pdf (Accessed 21 December 2021).

17. de Carvalho-Filho MA, Tio RA, Steinert Y. Twelve tips for implementing a community of practice for faculty development. Med Teach. 2020;42(2):143–9. Available from: https://www.tandfonline.com/doi/abs/10.1080/0142159X.2018.1552782 (Accessed 21 December 2021).

18. Driessen E, van Tartwijk J, Dornan T. The self-critical doctor: Helping students become more reflective. Br Med J. 2008 April 10;336(7648):827–30. Available from: https://www.bmj.com/content/336/7648/827.short (Accessed 21 December 2021).

16

Family medicine placements

Apprenticeship learning

Elizabeth I. Lamb, Abdulaziz Al-Mahrezi, and Hugh Alberti

KEY LEARNING POINTS

- ■ Family medicine (FM) is an ideal setting for apprenticeship learning (AL).
- ■ AL supports the development, under supervision, of skills, knowledge, and professional identity in an authentic clinical environment.
- ■ Recognition of the educational role of the clinical supervisors in AL is important; time, training, and resources should be made available to them.
- ■ Active participation is the key element of learning in FM placements.
- ■ Role modelling is an important component of AL; those supervising trainees should be aware of their function as a role model and seek to do this positively.

Apprenticeship learning in FM

The bedrock of FM teaching in undergraduate curricula has been the placement of medical students, usually individually or in very small groups, with FM doctors in community settings. Whether acknowledged explicitly or not, these placements have been based on AL. The Oxford English Dictionary defines an apprentice as follows: "A learner of a craft, bound to serve, and entitled to instruction from, his or her employer for a specified period".

> AL is important in becoming a doctor, providing the opportunity for tacit knowledge, skills, and attitudes to be demonstrated by experts and learned through role modelling in practice settings.

Apprenticeship provides the opportunity for "legitimate peripheral participation,[1] supporting the development of professional identity by socialising into a

DOI: 10.1201/9781003325734-19

BOX 16.1 A CASE STUDY FROM THE SULTAN QABOOS UNIVERSITY, OMAN

The College of Medicine & Health Sciences established a FM department early in its development. This enabled students (intake 130/year) to rotate to FM, for five weeks in Junior and three weeks in Senior Clerkships across the University FM, and affiliated community, health centres. Originally, to expose them to different clinical settings, students rotated as small groups (five to seven) spending a week in each health centre. They were dissatisfied with the rotation. Evaluation across faculty, tutors, and students revealed lack of continuity, for students and tutors, as the problem. Student feedback improved considerably when they spent the whole placement in a single health centre. The FM rotation was voted one of the best in subsequent years!

---

community of professional learning and practice".[2] The AL model provides the opportunity to engage with patients in a safe clinical environment, balancing "learning to know with learning to care", whilst developing the attitudes and behaviours required to be a doctor.[3] A case study from Oman (Box 16.1) illustrates how students and tutors value a safe FM environment.

Benefits of apprenticeship learning

The apprenticeship model offers early immersion in clinical environments, enabling practical and applied knowledge acquisition. Students have early exposure to common medical presentations and can transition from observation of clinicians to participation, performance, and then independence under close supervision. Experience and time in authentic workplaces facilitate experiential learning in real-life clinical practice[4] (Chapter 19). Attending home visits, nursing home visits, and community-based services all provide AL opportunities. Patients are not only individuals but are embedded within families and communities. AL allows students to take part in holistic care of people within their situational contexts. Ideally, they can follow the patient's journey through primary to secondary care or community services and sometimes back to primary care again; this is a key component of Longitudinal Integrated Clerkships (Chapter 17) but can be undertaken even within shorter block placements.[5]

> Situational learning through apprenticeship supports students to understand the importance of holistic, person-centred care and how patients journey through healthcare systems.

AL safeguards patients, refines and develops trainees' skills in supportive environments, while exposing them to workplace culture and potential role models.[6] Students can witness real ethical dilemmas, navigate challenging situations, and learn communication and consultation skills. Community placements allow observation of professional behaviour across interprofessional healthcare teams. Supported by reflection, this enables students to develop their own professional identity and recognise that they are legitimate contributors to healthcare.[7]

> Situational learning through apprenticeship supports students to develop their own professional identity and understand how they contribute to healthcare.

Challenges of apprenticeship learning

Many clinicians are not trained in supervision and may feel inadequately prepared to fulfil this role.[8] This can lead to job dissatisfaction and directly impact on the quality of the student's experience. Continuity of supervision can prove challenging in short clinical placements with large numbers of students. Offering "teach the teacher support" through professional development workshops for junior and senior clinicians, along with supervision and incentives to teach, can mitigate these challenges.

> Relationship and trust are important to facilitate meaningful feedback for apprentices.

Meaningful feedback can be supported through small student groups partaking in longitudinal placements in one setting (Box 16.1). When supervisors have responsibility for workplace-based competency sign offs, the relationship between supervisor and student risks becoming assessment focused. This may lead to a sense of formality, detracting from the authentic clinical experience. Offering mentorship to build relationships which focus not on assessment, but on students' professional identity development is important. Professional identity development has been highlighted as a key component of primary care placements post-COVID.[9]

> Create a cultural expectation of FM mentoring relationships which shift the focus from assessment to supporting personal professional development.

Workload and tensions between service provision and training present further challenges, particularly as patients correctly take priority. In poorly resourced and pressurised settings, training may be sidelined. Potential solutions include protected time in job plans for training and attending teacher support sessions.

In Oman, limited space in the university health centre has proved a significant barrier to effective AL, particularly as FM has an expanding residency training role. This barrier has been overcome by using both the university and community health centres as training sites. Undergraduates are exposed to two different learning

TABLE 16.1 Potential challenges and solutions in AL

Challenge	Solution
Teaching clinicians not formally trained	"Teach the Teacher" support and development programmes
Continuity of supervision	Long-term placements with a nominated supervisor
Focus of supervision on assessment	Assigning academic mentors with a remit of professional development not assessment
Tension between service provision and teaching	Protect time to teach, remunerate tutors appropriately
Lack of space for teaching	Utilise non-university health centres and other clinical team members

environments: one with more teaching and less workload; the other with less teaching but more clinical exposure. Efforts have been made to allow community health centre clinicians protected time to teach.

> Protected time to teach is key in facilitating AL.

Teaching methods have adapted in Oman to maximise AL. Initially, students took turns in clerking a patient in one room with a clinician. Now they are distributed across all consultation rooms broadening clinical exposure and with specific roles from observation to active participation. Though progress has been made, the nature of the short FM rotations means that workplace-based assessment remains the focus which has potential to interfere with clinical experience. Table 16.1 summarises the potential challenges and solutions in AL.

Cognitive apprenticeship learning in FM placements

In traditional AL models, students initially observe clinical practitioners and are then gradually entrusted with more tasks as they gain competency. In the cognitive apprenticeship model, teaching methods are highly specific and designed to enhance learning in clinical practice by making explicit the generally tacit cognitive processes of experts.[10] This helps students understand complex task performance, problem solve, reproduce procedures independently, and formulate their own personal learning goals. To promote situated learning within the cognitive model, six teaching approaches are proposed to help students acquire cognitive and meta-cognitive skills, focus their observation of expert performance in practice, and develop problem-solving skills.[11] These have been modified in Box 16.2 to contextualise them within FM placements.

BOX 16.2   FACILITATING LEARNING IN THE COGNITIVE APPRENTICESHIP MODEL

1. *Modelling:* Allow students to sit in surgeries. Actively demonstrate and explain skills and procedures they observe.

2. *Coaching:* Observe students undertaking part or whole consultations. Offer specific feedback on performance.

3. *Scaffolding:* Tailor support to students' individual knowledge levels, reducing this as their competency increases. Move from observing history taking to examination, the entire consultation, and then consulting alone followed by a debrief.

4. *Articulation:* Use debriefing time to question the students on why and how they reached decisions, offering opportunities to ask questions.

5. *Reflection:* Encourage students to consider their strengths and weaknesses and ways to enhance their professional development.

6. *Exploration:* Support students to develop learning goals for new or repeated activities. Provide opportunities to achieve their goals within the placement.

In addition, evidence highlights the beneficial effects of a positive learning climate. Teachers can foster this by showing interest in students' learning and making them feel respected.

The six teaching methods of the cognitive apprenticeship model, alongside a positive learning climate, can helpfully facilitate good clinical learning and teaching in FM.

Active learning in FM placements

A key component of AL is active learning—moving quickly from observation to participation before consulting alone (Chapter 19).

Family medicine placements provide an ideal setting to involve students actively in patient care through shared and student-led consultations.

In FM, students experience many patient interactions, a huge variety of presentations, and, most importantly, undifferentiated problems to strengthen their clinical reasoning skills. Students should move quickly from observing to leading consultations themselves, either with or without tutor observation. Box 16.3 contains tips to support student learning on FM placements.

Student-led consultations, or parallel surgeries, where students consult undifferentiated patients alone before debriefing with the tutor, are ideal for relatively experienced students. Tutors should be close by and available to review the patient,

---

BOX 16.3 IMPROVING STUDENT PARTICIPATION IN APPRENTICESHIP LEARNING

- Ensure students participate in consultations with all members of the primary healthcare team.
- In specific clinics (e.g. diabetes), ask students to connect the underpinning science and clinical knowledge with patients' presentations and management.
- Ideally sit in a triangle so that the student is actively involved in the consultation.
- Ask students to observe how clinicians interact with patients and their teams, the professional attitudes and skills demonstrated, and any behaviours they would wish to emulate.
- Use every opportunity to enable students to speak with patients and develop their communication and consultation skills.
- Explore opportunities for students to follow up patients in the clinic or through primary, secondary, and community care.

---

ideally with the student, after the student consultation. Evaluation of parallel consulting has shown this develops students' consulting and clinical reasoning skills.[12]

Teachers require time to teach and provide feedback. This can be dependent on delivery logistics which should be planned carefully. Students should be instructed on how to maximise gain from learning experiences and always given opportunity to debrief. In addition, students need "developmental space" (Chapter 19), i.e. sufficient intellectual space and time, to make sense and meaning of patient encounters.

> Students value and learn from the freedom and responsibility of taking the role of "the doctor" and, as long as patient safety is not compromised, should be given as much independence as possible.

Role modelling

Learning through close observation of others, role modelling, is a powerful means of transmitting values and ways of interacting with patients and colleagues.[13] Through role modelling, areas of the formal, informal, and hidden curriculum are taught, including prescribing habits, doctor–patient relationships, and leadership skills (Chapter 13). Individuals learn from role models through an active process of engagement, appraisal, selection of behaviours which are relevant to them, and construction of knowledge from the experience.[14] Reflection is key to this process enabling incorporation of observed actions into the student's values and behaviours.

> Positive FM role models play a crucial part in shaping students as professionals and supporting individuals towards careers in FM.

Those acting as potential role models to students on FM placements should be aware of their influence, and consciously provide positive role modelling experiences. Negative role modelling, including witnessing denigration of FM, can have a profound impact on individuals, potentially deterring them from careers in the specialty.[15] However, individuals can still positively shape their own professional identity through reflection on negative experience.[16] There are key institutional barriers to effective role modelling, including organisational structures that encourage overwork, lack of support, and time for teaching and a culture that accepts inadequate patient care and poor team dynamics.[17,18]

It is important to seek to overcome these barriers. We make the following recommendations for educational institutions to support positive role modelling in FM:

- FM teachers should be aware of their potential influence as role models and seek to demonstrate positive attributes and behaviours in all settings.

- "Teach the Teacher" programmes should raise awareness of role modelling and support individuals to be positive ones.

- Relationships, trust, and time are important. Positive role modelling can be facilitated by adequate resources and time to teach.

- Denigration of FM must be highlighted at educational institutions and a zero-tolerance approach taken to "bashing" of the specialty by role models.

Box 16.4 offers guidance, adapted from Swanwick et al.,[13] on becoming a good role model

Conclusion

We share here the benefits and challenges we have experienced facilitating AL in Oman and the UK. FM provides an ideal setting for student apprenticeship. We suggest some practical positive steps our international colleagues can take to embed this in their medical school curricula.

BOX 16.4 HOW TO BE A GOOD ROLE MODEL: A GUIDE FOR FAMILY MEDICINE[13]

- Be positive and enthusiastic about what you do.
- Be compassionate, open, and human.
- Be analytical about your performance as a role model.
- Model reflective practice, encourage students to talk about their encounters with role models. If things go wrong, be prepared to reflect on this with them.
- Articulate your values, support trainees to understand their own values.
- Try and be explicit about behaviours you are role modelling.
- Be learner-centred. Seek to facilitate relationships with trainees.
- Allow time for discussion and debrief following clinical encounters.
- Demonstrate respectful behaviour towards colleagues.
- Make time for personal and professional development activity.
- Seek to improve your workplace culture and values.

References

1. Lave JW. Etienne. Situated learning: Legitimate peripheral participation. Cambridge England: Cambridge University Press; 1991.
2. Dornan T, Osler F. Apprenticeship and the new medical education. J R Soc Med. 2005;98(3):91–5.
3. Pearson D, Nicholson S. How to succeed on primary care and community placements. Hoboken, UK: John Wiley & Sons, Inc.; 2016.
4. Yardley S, Teunissen PW, Dornan T. Experiential learning: AMEE Guide no. 63. Med Teach. 2012;34(2):e102–e15.
5. Worley P, Couper I, Strasser R, Graves L, Cummings B-A, Woodman R, et al. A typology of longitudinal integrated clerkships. Med Educ. 2016;50(9):922–32.
6. Rassie K. The apprenticeship model of clinical medical education: Time for structural change. N Z Med J. 2017;130(1461):66–72.
7. Bartlett M, Rees EL, McKinley RK. 'Knowledge leech' to 'part of the team': Students' learning in rural communities of practice. Educ Prim Care. 2018;29(1):5–10.
8. Kilminster S, Cottrell D, Grant J, Jolly B. AMEE Guide no. 27: Effective educational and clinical supervision. Med Teach. 2007;29(1):2–19.
9. Cullum RJ, Shaughnessy A, Mayat NY, Brown ME. Identity in lockdown: Supporting primary care professional identity development in the COVID-19 generation. Educ Prim Care. 2020;31(4):200–4.
10. Stalmeijer RE, Dolmans DHJM, Wolfhagen IHAP, Scherpbier AJJA. Cognitive apprenticeship in clinical practice: Can it stimulate learning in the opinion of students? Adv Health Sci Educ Theory Pract. 2009;14(4):535–46.
11. Collins A, Brown JS, Newman SE. Cognitive apprenticeship: Teaching the craft of reading, writing and mathematics. Thinking J Philos Children. 1988;8(1):2–10.
12. Allan R, McAleer S. Parallel consulting method: Student and tutor evaluation in general practice. Educ Prim Care. 2021;32(5):308–10.
13. Swanwick T, Forrest K, O'Brien BC. Understanding medical education: Evidence, theory, and practice. Newark, UK: John Wiley & Sons, Inc.; 2019.
14. Passi V, Johnson N. The impact of positive doctor role modeling. Med Teach. 2016;38(11):1139–45.
15. Alberti H, Banner K, Collingwood H, Merritt K. 'Just a GP': A mixed method study of undermining of general practice as a career choice in the UK. BMJ Open. 2017;7(11):e018520.
16. Miettola J, Mäntyselkä P, Vaskilampi T. Doctor–patient interaction in Finnish primary health care as perceived by first year medical students. BMC Med Educ. 2005;5(1):34.
17. Cruess SR, Cruess RL, Steinert Y. Role modelling: Making the most of a powerful teaching strategy. BMJ. 2008;336(7646):718–21.
18. Lamb L, Burford B, Alberti H. The impact of role modelling on the future general practitioner workforce: A systematic review. Educ in Prim Care. 2022. doi: 10.1080/14739879.2022.2079097

17

Longitudinal integrated clerkships

Jill Konkin and Shrijana Shrestha

SUMMARY OF KEY LEARNING POINTS

■ Longitudinal integrated clerkships (LICs) are based on continuity of patient care, clinical teachers, and learning environments to ensure a relationship-centred clerkship model.

■ Centring an LIC in family medicine (FM) is an ideal context for introducing LICs into the undergraduate curriculum using various LIC models adapted to rural or urban settings.

■ LIC models depend on context. Rural settings offer continuous, fully immersive attachments to follow patients over time. Adapting to urban settings can be more challenging.

■ Learners in LICs become valued members of local healthcare teams, spend more time "in the role of a physician", and develop an enhanced sustained patient-centred approach.

■ It is important for urban medical schools to introduce FM-based LICs to enable students to understand a generalist approach to healthcare beyond specialist-based tertiary care.

■ The continuity of student LIC attachments increases satisfaction for patients and clinical teachers.

What are longitudinal integrated clerkships?

LICs are established clerkship models that have been implemented in many countries. The first of these clerkships was at the University of Minnesota, USA, in 1971. The LICs took hold in Australia in the 1990s and then spread more widely in the early 2000s.

In an LIC, medical students spend an extended period of time in one clinical setting or several linked clinical settings. LICs are based on continuity principles

DOI: 10.1201/9781003325734-20

initially described by Hirsh et al.[1] and expanded by Hudson et al.[2] The three foundational continuity principles are as follows:

1. Continuity of patient care
2. Continuity with clinical teachers
3. Continuity of learning environment (students are in the same placements throughout the length of the LIC)

Members of a newly established Consortium of Longitudinal Integrated Clerkship (CLIC) met in 2007. The group affirmed the first two continuity principles as a definitional statement and added "meet the majority of the year's core clinical competencies across multiple disciplines simultaneously".[3]

Continuity principles are foundational to LICs.

Worley et al.[4] identified three broad categories of LICs: amalgamative, blended, and comprehensive. The study that produced this paper was undertaken because "what defines an LIC is often contentious outside the LIC community".[4] With ad hoc definitions, it is very difficult to undertake studies and comparisons across programmes. The LIC types were distinguished by length of programme, number of disciplines across the academic year covered, and presence or absence of block rotations (see Box 17.1).

Given that Cluster A did not meet the "majority criterion in the CLIC definition in regard to either curriculum time or curriculum content",[4] it was proposed that these programmes "should not be referred to as LICs but should rather be described as 'Amalgamative Clerkships' (ACs)".[4]

LICs can be classified into three delivery models based on length, disciplines covered, and presence or absence of additional block rotations.

BOX 17.1 CATEGORIES OF LICs[4]

Cluster	Type	Length: % of academic year	Disciplines covered/year	External rotations
A	Amalgamative	Less than 50%	2+ but less than 50% of total	None
B	Blended	50–89%	Majority	Complementary block rotations
C	Comprehensive	90–100%	All	Most have none but there may be short burst experiences connected to curriculum

It is well-established that LIC students perform as well as or, in some cases, better than their peers who remain in rotation-based clerkships (RBCs).[5] Students placed in LICs are in one clinical environment or in a connected series of the same learning environments at the same time every week for the duration of the clerkship. This allows the development of longitudinal therapeutic relationships with patients and educational relationships with teachers. In a multi-programme study, Hauer[6] et al. found that LIC students described being integrated into their healthcare teams and functioning in a "doctor-like role" in contrast to RBC students who described a student-like role of filling gaps with a less authentic role in patient care. LIC students become more patient-centered through their clerkship year in contrast to RBC students and this is sustained beyond the clerkship year.[7]

The rural LIC model allows students to experience continuity of care through longitudinal relationships with patients, teachers, and healthcare teams.

While LICs can be implemented in any setting, for those medical educators wanting to increase the number of graduates who choose generalist careers, in particular FM, and especially those who are wanting to contribute to the workforce in rural and remote areas, the context in which an LIC is implemented is important. Bates and Ellaway state:

"Individual attitudes and the resulting behaviours and the development of physician identities can be highly dependent on the contexts within which they are developed and will continue to influence future practice."[8]

Rural and small urban community LICs do graduate more generalist physicians including, but not limited to, family physicians.[9,10] There are successful urban LICs, though adapting to non-rural contexts can be more challenging, especially if the goal is to encourage more students to pursue FM.[11]

In the setting of a lower middle income country (LMIC) like Nepal, a few medical schools have LICs in their undergraduate curricula either as a part of community-based medical education or as a placement in primary level health facility, community, or district hospitals.[12] These are generally Cluster A (amalgamative) or Cluster B (blended) LIC models. However, unlike most LICs in the west, these usually apply to the whole class, not just small cohorts and are mandatory not voluntary. The duration varies from a few weeks to six months.

Such placements not only help students understand continuity of care but will also prepare them to work in resource-poor settings and understand the role of a doctor and community expectations in that context. Such placements under the supervision of a family physician familiarise them with holistic patient care in contrast to the specialty and subspecialty-based fragmented care at a large urban teaching hospital. Benefits of LICs are not simply for learners. Both patients and clinical teachers report increased satisfaction with their continuity relationships with LIC students.[13,14]

Ensuring family medicine is a core discipline in LICs is key for influencing career choice in primary care.

Establishing an LIC

There are several resources to assist with the development of LICs.[3,15]
    Key steps:

1. Determine intended learning outcome(s) of the LIC.

2. Choose the LIC administrative team (clerkship coordinator, administrator, possibly a learning specialist, and programme evaluator) and identify funding sources.

3. Identify champions in the undergraduate medical education leadership team and bring them on board early.

4. Build a development and implementation team to include the clinical teachers for the LIC.

5. Identify the cluster type that is possible in the current undergraduate medical programme and where the LIC will be situated.

6. Determine how the LIC will meet the three continuity principles.

7. Determine the requirements for sites, e.g. patient flow, breadth of local health services and availability of local teachers for rural LICs, and core specialty discipline leads for urban LICs, which need to include FM.

8. For rural LICs, determine the information communication technologies needed to support learners distant from the urban campuses of most medical schools.

9. For rural LICs, accommodations for students and logistics, such as getting them to and from their rural sites, in particular in LMICs, need to be part of the initial and ongoing planning.

Enablers and challenges

In many high-resource countries, there has been a long tradition of distributed medical education which is defined loosely as the practice of situating medical education outside of the Academic Health Sciences Centres associated with North American medical schools.[16] In both North America and globally, this has primarily referred to medical education programmes that are situated outside of the urban home of the medical school.

This has developed a cohort of experienced rural physician teachers that have been invaluable to the implementation of rural LICs. Many governments in these countries have identified the need to increase the rural and remote workforce, so they have developed initiatives supporting rural medical education. These initiatives have provided funds to support learners and teachers in distributed programmes, including LICs.

A significant challenge for generalist and, in particular, rural generalist LICs has been the geographical narcissism[17] of urban faculties of medicine and the overvaluing of subspecialty medicine. These are manifest in many ways starting with the view that physician teachers in the community aren't as good as subspecialists in tertiary settings and that community settings do not have the breadth nor the type of clinical presentations required to meet the objectives for the year that the LIC covers. Until recently, the culture of medical schools has been immersed in tertiary care subspecialty medicine, so pre-clerkship students have a significant fear that they will miss something if they undertake an LIC of any type (Chapter 6).

This latter is mitigated when all students in a medical school are required to complete a year-long LIC but many faculties of medicine have LICs for a small cohort of their class. Some of the newer medical schools developed with a social accountability mandate plus a few more established medical schools who have reoriented to social accountability have a more generalist base, but there are not yet sufficient of these to make a difference to the crisis in FM workforce around the world (Chapter 3).

Common to all LICs in communities distant from the medical school are issues with logistics. In many countries, the rural and remote workforce is stretched thin and has significant turnover. LICs, especially Cluster C, need communities with a stable core of clinical teachers as well as a broad range of services, both in the community and in the hospital. For programmes shorter than one year, accommodation for learners can be a barrier. Transportation can also be problematic for some programmes.

> Communities with a broad range of primary and secondary care services and a stable core of clinical teachers are well placed to deliver LICs.

LICs that are widely distributed need administrative support that is different from that required for RBCs. Information communication technology can be a barrier, including the absence of stable internet and platforms that are inappropriate for distributed communities of learning. Urban decision-makers are often reticent to recognise these resource needs and are loathe to distribute resources, both personnel and financial, even when they are willing to send learners to distributed sites. These barriers are more pronounced in LMICs where government support is not as robust.

Urban programmes struggle with the specialist siloes which make continuity and integration harder to achieve. These programmes also struggle to integrate community and primary care with secondary and tertiary care in a seamless way. For urban programmes wanting to instil a generalist approach plus generalist skills in their learners and/or to increase the number of generalist graduates, the challenge is to have students learning in a generalist environment with generalists for a significant part of their LIC. Generalists in all of the core disciplines of the clerkship year will need to be recruited as the primary teachers.

Conclusion: Why is this important for family medicine and primary care?

LICs that have family physicians as the predominant teachers will increase the numbers of graduates who chose this specialty and other generalist specialties. Those that integrate community-based and hospital-based care afford learners a more holistic understanding of the practice of medicine.

All LICs will increase the patient-centredness of their graduates and an understanding of the value of continuity of care. Learners in these programmes will benefit from the advantages of having teachers who know them and follow their growth over time. In high-resource countries, many medical schools have turned to rural LICs as an important initiative to increase the number of generalist physicians, in particular rural generalists, that graduate from their programmes.

LICs offer the opportunity to bridge the gap between primary and secondary care clinically and educationally and prepare students for a world of evolving healthcare.

In countries like Nepal, graduates of the medical schools become eligible for a licence for independent practice immediately after completing their undergraduate programme and could be posted to any peripheral health facility where they may not have direct supervision from more experienced physicians. These postings call for leadership skills, team spirit, good decision-making, and the ability to mobilise resources and engage the community. An LIC which places students at primary-level health facilities/district hospitals ensures these competencies in graduates. These skills and abilities are necessary for learners in high-resource countries in order to work in smaller communities. Participants in LICs become competently confident about their ability to work in all settings.*

If we focus on present-day healthcare delivery systems and their existing gaps in care for individual patients and their communities in countries worldwide, the shift of patient care from single disease and acute illness models to providing holistic care for people and bridging the gap between primary and secondary care requires a whole new approach. LICs can be one of the initiatives in alignment with such an approach.[18]

References

1. Hirsh DA, Ogur B, Thibault G, Cox E. "Continuity" as an organizing principle for clinical education reform. N Engl J Med. 2007;356:858–66.
2. Hudson JN, Poncelet AN, Weston K, Bushnell JA, Farmer EA. Longitudinal integrated clerkships. Med Teach. 2017;39(1):7–13. doi: 10.1080/0142159X.2017.1245855
3. Alliance for Clinical Education. Poncelet A, Hirsh D (eds.), Longitudinal integrated clerkships: Principles, outcomes, practical tools, and future directions. North Syracuse NY: Gegensatz Press; 2016.
4. Worley P, Couper I, Strasser R et al. A typology of longitudinal integrated clerkships. Med Educ. 2016;50:922–32.
5. Walters l, Greenhill J, Richards J, Ward H, Campbell N, Ash J, Schuwirth LWT. Outcomes of longitudinal integrated clinical placements for students, clinicians and society. Med Educ. 2012;46:1028–41.
6. Hauer KE, Hirsh D, Ma I, Hansen L, Ogur B, Poncelet AN, Alexander EK, O'Brien BC. The role of role: Learning in longitudinal integrated and traditional block clerkships. Med Educ. 2012;46:698–710.

7. Gaufberg E, Hirsh D, Krupat E, Ogur B, Pelletier S, Reiff D, Bor D. Into the future: Patient-centredness endures in longitudinal integrated clerkship graduates. Med Educ. 2014;48(6):572–82.

8. Bates J, Ellaway RH. Mapping the dark matter of context: A conceptual scoping review. Med Educ. 2016;50:807–16.

9. Halaas GW, Zink T, Finstad D, Bollin K, Center B. Recruitment and retention of rural physicians: Outcomes from the Rural Physician Associate Program of Minnesota. J Rural Health. 2008;24:345–52.

10. Tao A Poncelet AN, Lemoine D, Konkin J, Wamsley M, Mazotti L, Sullivan J, Teherani A, Ziv T, Riegels NS. Longitudinal integrated clerkship graduates: Practice trends over a 13-year period. 2019. Poster Presented at Consortium of Longitudinal Integrated Clerkships Annual Conference, Vancouver BC.

11. Richards E, Elliott L, Jackson B, Panesar A. Longitudinal integrated clerkship evaluations in UK medical schools: A narrative literature review. Educ Prim Care. 2022;33(3):148–55. doi: 10.1080/14739879.2021.2021809

12. Marahatta SB, Sinha NP, Dixit H, Shrestha IB, Pokharel PK. Comparative study of community medicine practice in MBBS curriculum of health institutions of Nepal. Kathmandu Univ Med J. 2009;7(4):461–69.

13. Hudson JN, Knight PJ, Weston KM. Patient perceptions of innovative longitudinal integrated clerkships based in regional, rural and remote primary care: A qualitative study. BMC Family Pract. 2012;13:72. doi: 10.1186/1471-2296-13-72

14. Walters L, Prideaux D, Worley P, Greenhill J. Demonstrating the value of longitudinal integrated placements to general practice preceptors. Med Educ. 2011;45(5):455–63.

15. Ellaway R, Graves L, Berry S, Myhre D, Cummings B-A, Konkin J. Twelve tips for designing and running longitudinal integrated clerkships. Med Teach. 2013;35(12):989–95.

16. Ellaway R, Bates J. Distributed medical education in Canada. Can Med Educ J. 2018;9(1):e1–e5..

17. Fors M. Geographical narcissism in psychotherapy: Countermapping urban assumptions about power, space, and time. Psychoanal Psychol. 2018;35(4):446–53. doi: 10.1037/pap0000179

18. Bartlett M, Muir F. A new model of undergraduate clinical education. Br J Gen Pract. 2018;68:216–17.

18

Interprofessional learning

Nynke Scherpbier and Carmen Ka Man Wong

SUMMARY OF KEY LEARNING POINTS

- Collaborative practice is essential for the evolving complexities of healthcare; this highlights the importance of interprofessional learning (IPL).
- Competencies for interprofessional working include communication, role clarification, teamwork, individual/family/community-centred care, leadership, and conflict management.
- Sociocultural constructivism, Kolb's learning cycle, and the Kirkpatrick model of evaluation can help design individual and group learning activities.
- Implementation of IPL requires organisational commitment, support, and faculty development.
- Family medicine (FM) educators are in a unique position to be key advocators, leaders, and role models in IPL.

Defining interprofessional learning

IPL is the development of the ability to work collaboratively with other professionals and disciplines.[1] The definition of professionals is wide ranging, extending from core healthcare professionals, e.g. primary care physicians, nurses, physiotherapists, dieticians, pharmacists, psychologists, and occupational therapists, to other providers supporting care, e.g. administrators and managers.

Interprofessional collaboration occurs when multiple health professionals, of differing skill backgrounds and disciplines, provide a comprehensive service to deliver high-quality care by working with patients, families, carers, and communities.[2] Interprofessional education occurs when students from two or more professions learn about from, and with, each other to enable effective collaboration and improve health outcomes.[3] IPL is a lifelong continuum from undergraduate through to

DOI: 10.1201/9781003325734-21

continuous professional development. It is a prerequisite for a collaborative practice-ready health workforce.

Patients are increasingly presenting to family doctors with multiple comorbid conditions and complex social needs. There is an urgent need for effective interprofessional collaboration, with expert input from multiple professionals, to tailor management and preventative interventions. Interprofessional care teams are essential to navigate the increasing complexities of healthcare systems, interagency financing, and to identify appropriate local health and community resources for optimising patient care.

In 2008, an international environmental survey of IPL practices in 42 countries, when defining the educational benefits of IPL, used input from multiple professionals in their local healthcare contexts exploring their real-world experience and insights.[2] They identified health policy benefits which included improvements in workplace practices, productivity, patient outcomes, safety, and staff morale.

Thus, IPL should be seen as not just a component but as a key process in improving the efficiency and effectiveness of primary healthcare services and patient outcomes. Educators and policymakers should explore the opportunities offered by multidisciplinary care teams and take advantage of the positive impact of IPL.

> The need for interprofessional collaboration is growing due to the complexity of healthcare demands. IPL is key to improving interprofessional collaboration.

Challenges to interprofessional learning and collaborative practice

Every healthcare environment is unique. Local and regional diversity, unmet health needs, cultural contexts, and structural organisational differences shape this unicity. Interdisciplinary and collaborative practice must address local needs and challenges. Although healthcare professionals may engage with a range of professionals and disciplines, they are not necessarily adequately prepared, or have the essential skills, knowledge, and values, to practise collaboratively.[4] Professions form their own unique culture of language, habits, and customs. These lead to differing values and norms, making them vulnerable to prejudice and difficulties in understanding and communication.[5]

The skills required to work collaboratively within a team and resolve interprofessional conflicts include effective communication, clarity about boundaries of roles and responsibilities, recognition of weaknesses, and the ability to pre-empt problems. There are many competency frameworks for interprofessional collaboration. The Canadian Interprofessional Health Collaborative framework, for example, defines essential competency domains to inform attitudes, behaviours, values, and judgements for collaborative practice[6] (see Box 18.1).

> For effective interprofessional collaboration and team working, a broad spectrum of competencies should be acquired to develop clear understanding of each other's roles.

> **BOX 18.1 COMPETENCY FRAMEWORK FOR INTERPROFESSIONAL COLLABORATION[6]**
>
> - Role clarification
> - Team functioning
> - Interprofessional communication
> - Patient/client/family/ community-centred care
> - Interprofessional conflict resolution
> - Collaborative leadership

Approaches to interprofessional learning

Theories on IPL delivery commonly focus on cognition, sociocultural constructivism, intergroup processes, and power.[7] Learning through sociocultural constructivism occurs when students interact not only with the instructional material but also with professional groups in interprofessional environments, and by sharing and debriefing with peers. Learning is thus contextual and reflective. Students are able to appreciate established and alternative perspectives on healthcare and on collective, group, and individual professional philosophies.[7]

Learning domains can translate to undergraduate or postgraduate teaching and learning outcomes based on the competencies required for collaborative practice[6] (see Table 18.1).

Cognition and knowledge are actively constructed. Interprofessional education focuses on using diverse activities to address different learning styles, either individual or predominant within a profession. Providing opportunities for interaction is important. In addition to in-person or online lectures, experiential learning is essential. It

TABLE 18.1 Example of interprofessional learning domains and learning outcomes

Domain	Learning outcome (examples)
1. Teamwork	• Ability to be both team leader and team member • Knowledge of team dynamics and barriers to teamwork
2. Roles and responsibilities	• Knowledge of own professional role, responsibilities, and expertise • Knowledge of other professional roles, responsibilities, and expertise
3. Communication	• Active listening and expressing own knowledge and expertise competently to different professions • Negotiating a joint care plan
4. Learning and critical reflection	• Critically reflecting on own performance and relationship with others
5. Relationship with, and recognising the needs of the patient	• Effective engagement with patient, family carers, and communities • Collaborative care planning with multiple professionals
6. Ethical practice	• Acknowledge each professional views and opinions are equally valid and important • Foster IPL culture at work

offers the opportunity for application and reflection (Chapter 19). Concrete experiences, e.g. interviews, attachments, visits, and simulations, supported by Kolb's experiential learning cycle, enhance critical reflection, abstract thinking, and problem-solving.[8] Intentionally crafted team-based learning interactions, e.g. group discussions, team tasks, shared individuals and collective reflections, and project-based assignments, help participants engage with content and, importantly, each other. Careful consideration is crucial to ensure the instructional material and active group learning activities, based on critical thinking and reflection, align with the intended learning outcomes.

> Diverse, interactive, experiential IPL opportunities need to be carefully designed to align with the intended learning outcomes.

An important aspect of interprofessional collaboration and education is the presence of power. Power dynamics always exist in interprofessional collaboration, but not necessarily in a negative sense. It is important that learners recognise power dynamics, hidden agendas and their impacts, and build a respectful collaborative culture. Social network theory, i.e. the study of people, organisations, and their interactions, can help make power dynamics visible. Examining the social constructs underpinning roles and responsibilities, formal and informal relationships, individuals and their interactions can expose the strong ties and dynamics potentially affecting the network and team working.[9]

Key learning opportunities for interprofessional collaboration include transitions in care, case conferences, and quality of healthcare pathways and planning. The intended learning can have a particular focus such as medication management. Reflection with, and feedback from, facilitators help students understand the dynamics, strengths, and shortfalls of the healthcare system and collaborative processes.

> The design and implementation of interprofessional education needs underpinning with the relevant educational theories. Power dynamics should be acknowledged.

Implementation and evaluation

Implementation of IPL at undergraduate and postgraduate levels requires an action plan. Key steps in implementation are detailed in Box 18.2.

During implementation, there are practical considerations for both the organisation and the curriculum (see Table 18.2). These include faculty/organisational support, content development, core teaching, and learning principles.

Professions and disciplines are traditionally organised in silos and delivered through specific, relatively isolated, training streams. This leads, in both undergraduate and postgraduate environments, to potential barriers to IPL implementation. To develop the necessary interactive learning, education faculty leads from *all* the involved

---

BOX 18.2 ACTIONS FOR IMPLEMENTATION OF INTERPROFESSIONAL LEARNING AND EDUCATION

1. Agree to common vision and purpose for IPL with key stakeholders across all faculties and organisations.
2. Develop IPL curricula.
3. Provide organisational support for development and delivery.
4. Introduce IPL into all undergraduate and postgraduate programmes.
5. Ensure staff training and competency in developing, delivering, and evaluating programmes.
6. Ensure continuous commitment to IPL.

---

professions must join to contribute. This can be challenging for onsite professionals who may normally have limited interaction.

Implementation can be further complicated by the logistical constraints of scheduling, space, staffing capacity, funding, and the relatively complex content. A steering group of core educators from each profession or discipline can help clarify and solve the challenges and sensitivities and support engagement with senior leadership for endorsement and practical resources. Interprofessional competencies must be developed through a shared common professional goal with unified outcomes and integrated processes. An approach based on parallel professionally siloed processes does not work and must be avoided.

Given the wide-ranging impact that IPL can have on patients, family, and communities as well as professionals, evaluation should be considered early, before

TABLE 18.2 Practical considerations for implementation of interprofessional learning and education

---

Practical considerations

Organisational

- Develop a taskforce with representation from the different professions involved.
- Seek senior leadership commitment and institutional support.
- List organisation support in terms of human and financial resources.
- Develop learning strategy for education and training and in daily practice.
- Identify individual and departmental champions and advocates.
- Ensure staff training to build interprofessional learning culture serving students across professions that are different from that of the individual staff member.

Curricular

- Develop shared objectives with interpretation relevant to the profession.
- Co-construct programme content from scratch with different professions.
- Develop well-constructed learning outcomes that delineate knowledge, skills, attitudes, and behaviour.
- Utilise diverse learning methods to cater to different learning styles.
- Contextualise learning with real-world experience and insights and group interaction.
- Design assessments to include individual and group projects, tasks, and reflection.
- Align scheduling, logistics, and coordination.
- Seek technical and administrative support.

---

implementation. It must be well- planned from the outset. For IPL and training, mixed modes of evaluation can incorporate pre- and post-surveys and quantitative surveys such as the Role Performance Questionnaire,[10] Readiness for Interprofessional Learning Scale,[11] and the Interdisciplinary Education Perception Scale.[12] Kirkpatrick's model of educational outcomes provides a useful framework. It evaluates beyond the knowledge, skills, and attitudes acquired by learners to explore behavioural changes in a student's healthcare practice and aspires to identify outcomes and impact for patients, family, and communities.[13] The call to provide evidence on the impact of IPL on patient outcomes is legitimate. However, this is hard to realise given the broad scope of variables involved in IPL interventions. Dissemination and active sharing of findings with stakeholders across multiple professions can help enhance the IPL culture and instigate further improvements in learning and training programmes.

> IPL implementation requires more planning and effort than uniprofessional education. All the professionals involved must have a common shared goal and unified outcomes.

Change management

Apart from organisational and educational structural processes, challenges may arise higher up in the healthcare system from lack of collaborative practice within the faculty or healthcare environment. It is important to recognise that there are wider influences and processes at play. These include challenges such as the structural environment, the design of interactive and collaborative spaces, and intangible factors such as working cultures or shared decision-making processes. These can impact on communication strategies across professions and require different approaches to conflict management. In addition, institutional support in terms of governance models, personnel policies, operating procedures, protocols, and practices may affect change management.

When negotiating a shared goal and plan for IPL, it is crucial to devote time to exploring the different stakeholder perspectives and the required policies and procedures. At a macro-level, the planning, commissioning, and financing of services influence how health and educational systems work together. The formal tasks and responsibilities across healthcare professionals can vary between countries and lead to different collaborative constructions.[2,14]

FM academics have important roles in research, teaching, administration, and leadership (Chapter 5). They can impact significantly as catalysts to motivate governmental support for progressing IPL. Improving the ecosystem of collaborative practice can impact on education and help resolve barriers to IPL.[14]

> The sustainable success of interprofessional education depends on changes at higher system levels. FM academics can be important catalysts to achieving this.

Advocacy and leadership in family medicine

FM with its holistic view of person-centred medicine provides an excellent environment to learn about collaborative work within the primary care team and how care is coordinated between professionals. FM educators are ideal advocates for collaborative practice and are key leaders in carrying out IPL. Given inherent differences in healthcare systems, cultural contexts, and educational arenas, the starting point for IPL programmes will be different. It requires a strong understanding of the resources available to promote change. FM is well placed to see the healthcare system from a bird's-eye perspective and build an understanding of how care providers relate to each other.[15] This advantage places FM in an excellent position to pioneer IPL endeavours.

> FM with its holistic person-centred and primary care team–based approach is in an ideal position to facilitate IPL.

Conclusion

The evolving complexity of healthcare, delivered across health and social sectors within local contexts and constraints, demands effective collaborative working. IPL is an important prerequisite to producing a collaborative practice-ready workforce. It should be mandatory training for professions, disciplines, and skilled workers in the healthcare arena. Medical educators should be active advocates of IPL. FM educators are in a prime position to role model collaborative learning and interprofessional working in education and practice.

References

1. Miller R, Scherpbier N, van Amsterdam L, Guedes V, Pype P. Inter-professional education and primary care: EFPC position paper. Prim Health Care Res Dev. 2019;20:e138. doi: 10.1017/S1463423619000653.
2. World Health Organisation. WHO/HRH/HPN/10.3: Framework for action on interprofessional education and collaborative practice. Geneva: WHO Press; 2010.
3. World Health Organisation. WHO/HIS/SDS/2015.20: WHO global strategy on people-centred and integrated health services. Geneva: WHO Press; 2015.
4. Zaudke J, Paolo A, Kleoppel J, Phillips C, Shrader S. The impact of an interprofessional practice experience on readiness for interprofessional learning. Fam Med. 2016;48:371–6.
5. Hall P. Interprofessional teamwork: Professional cultures as barriers. J Interprof Care. 2005;19(Suppl. 1):188–96. doi: 10.1080/13561820500081745
6. Canadian Interprofessional Health Collaborative. Canadian Interprofessional Health Collaborative (CIHC) framework. Available from: https://www.mcgill.ca/ipeoffice/ipe-curriculum/cihc-framework (Accessed 15 June 2022).
7. Hean S, Green C, Anderson E, Morris D, John C, Pitt R, O'Halloran C. The contribution of theory to the design, delivery, and evaluation of interprofessional curricula: BEME Guide no. 49. Med Teach. 2018;40(6):542–58.

8. Kolb D. Experiential learning: Experience as the source of learning and development (Vol. 1). New Jersey: Prentice Hall; 1984. doi: 10.1080/0142159X.2018.1432851

9. Nimmon L, Artino AR Jr, Varpio L. Social network theory in interprofessional education: Revealing hidden power. J Grad Med Educ. 2019;11(3):247–50. doi: 10.4300/JGME-D-19-00253.1

10. Kinner N, Roche AM, Freeman T, Addy D. Responding to alcohol and other drug issues: The effect of role adequacy and role legitimacy on motivation and satisfaction. Drugs: Educ Prev Policy. 2005;12(6):449–63.

11. Mattick K, Bligh J. Readiness for interprofessional learning scale. In: Bluteau P, Jackson A. (eds.), Interprofessional education making it happen. Hampshire: Palgrave Macmillan; 2009. pp. 125–142.

12. McFadyen AK, Maclaren WM, Webster VS. The interdisciplinary education perception scale (IEPS): An alternative remodelled sub-scale structure and its reliability. J Interprof Care. 2007;21(4):433–43. doi: 10.1080/13561820701352531

13. Kirkpatrick D. Great ideas revisited. Train Dev J. 1996;50:54–57.

14. Ho K, Borduas F, Frank B et al. Facilitating the integration of interprofessional education into quality health care: Strategic roles of academic institutions; 2006. Available from: https://www.researchgate.net/publication/237476918_Facilitating_the_Integration_of_Interprofessional_Education_into_Quality_Health_Care_Strategic_Roles_of_Academic_Institutions (Accessed 15 June 2022)

15. Larivaara P, Taanila A. Towards interprofessional family-oriented teamwork in primary services: The evaluation of an education programme. J Interpro Care. 2004;18(2):153–63. doi: 10.1080/13561820410001686918.

Teaching and learning
Methodologies

No bubble is so iridescent or floats longer than that blown by the successful teacher.

William Osler

Experiential learning for undergraduate medical students

Thandaza Cyril Nkabinde and Julia Blitz

SUMMARY OF KEY LEARNING POINTS

- Students need exposure to experiences that enable them to build on pre-existing knowledge as they develop competence.
- Experiential learning requires students to engage in authentic activities and reflective practice about their learning.
- Self-regulation is a critical skill in professional lifelong learning that enables recognition of what needs to be learnt and develops agency in achieving that.
- Educators can create an environment that encourages student agency for their own learning and supports students to use the feedback they receive.
- Experiential learning is deepened when students develop cultural humility that enriches their context-specific sociocultural interactions.

Defining experiential learning

Experiential learning is defined as "the ability of the student to construct knowledge and meaning learnt in the classroom to real life experiences they participate in".[1] A crucial component of this learning is reflection. Through this, they realise the process of "learning by doing" which enables them to learn and build specific competencies.[2] Creating experiential learning opportunities enables students to participate in tasks and gain competencies, whilst building on pre-existing knowledge.[3]

> Experiential learning is the process of learning that occurs through reflection on doing.

DOI: 10.1201/9781003325734-23

Kolb's experiential learning theory

Kolb's experiential learning theory (Figure 19.1) introduces a learning cycle which explains how students' experiences from their external world (concrete experience) are brought into their private world of thought and emotions (reflective observation). This allows them to interpret these experiences, by giving them personal meaning (abstract conceptualisation), leading to planning of new actions in response to the interpretations (active experimentation).[4,5]

In practice, students may start the cycle at different points of entry. It is therefore critical that the clinical educator guides the student through this cycle of learning.

Medical education has a strong history of "learning on the job", a concept well underpinned by experiential learning theory, which suggests that learning may be triggered by experiences.[1] As students meet different learning tasks, they have the opportunity to be reflective and identify difference(s) between this new experience and their prior knowledge and past encounters (Mezirow's disorienting dilemma—see later). This enables them to adapt to the realisation of these differences.[6] The medical educator can guide this process, to ensure the student moves towards achieving their learning outcomes and becoming a professional. By mastering reflection on, and learning from, their experiences, they can refine their approach to new tasks to meet new future challenges.

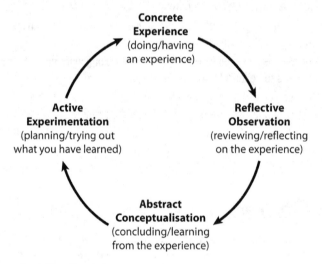

FIGURE 19.1 Kolb's experiential learning cycle.

How can you encourage reflective practice?

Reflecting on experiences to improve professional practice is an important attribute of a healthcare professional's lifelong learning.[7] Gibbs reflective cycle (Figure 19.2) is a useful tool for encouraging this. It assists students to plan a way forward based on their clinical experiences.[8]

The tool has six stages—"describing", "feeling", "evaluation", "analysis", "conclusion", and "action plan". To achieve the full potential of reflective practice, the educator

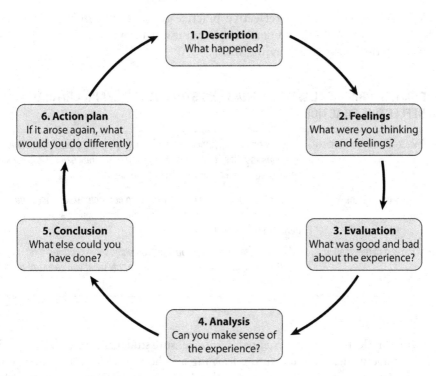

FIGURE 19.2 Gibbs reflective cycle (1988).[8]

assists the student through all stages, ensuring an action plan is reached. This may involve posing questions at each stage (see Figure 19.2) to encourage deep reflection.

> Reflection is a vehicle that can encourage lifelong improvement of professional practice.

Writing a reflective journal, using the Gibbs reflective cycle, is one best way to get students interacting with reflective practice. This enables educators to engage with students on a 1:1 basis, thus debriefing the encounter and facilitating learning. An initial prompt may be: *"Recently you have had encounters (concrete experiences) that have affected you in different ways (reflective observation). Using the Gibbs reflective cycle, consider how you might respond/act differently should this occur again"*.

Experiential educational activities are designed for transformative student learning. Mezirow's model of transformative learning suggests that students' baseline belief systems or frameworks may be challenged by new encounters.[6] By reflecting on their previous perceptions and understanding, they can modify their initial understanding and make new meaning. This should ultimately lead to why, what, and how they learn. Transformative learning enables individuals to learn from their experiences and move from one development level to another.

We encourage critically reflective practice throughout clinical exposure. The FM educator can help the students acquire transformative learning skills.[9] Box 19.1 shows practical ways of achieving this.

BOX 19.1   PRACTICAL WAYS OF ENABLING STUDENTS TO LEARN CRITICALLY REFLECTIVE PRACTICE

Prior to the clinical rotation	*"Reflect on prior experiences before engaging in the proposed clinical activities"* sensitising the student to possible hindrances/challenges they need to work on, encouraging learning to happen
Midway through the rotation	*"Reflect on your progress thus far, using concrete experiences that come to mind"*, asking them to reflect on their progress along their transformation journey
At the end of the rotation	*"What transformation do you feel took place for you during this rotation"* and particularly *"how will you apply what you've learnt to your future rotations"*?

Critical reflection and experiential learning ensure students are regularly sensitised to thinking about their past and future learning and how to self-regulate their learning. Self-regulation is defined as "a process that helps guide an individual's goal-directed activities, by controlling and managing their self-generated cognition (thoughts), affect (feelings), and behaviour (actions)."[10,11] This aligns with Bandura's social cognitive learning theory that learning takes place in social settings through observations and cognitive processes; learners make sense of what they see in order to choose what behaviour(s) to adopt.[12] As they progress through medical school, students need to learn self-regulation. In this way, they can show agency, by initiating and directing their own learning efforts, thus not just depending on their educators.[13]

Self-regulation of learning is critical for medical students, as they become lifelong learners.

Cultural humility: Orientating students to understand community culture

When planning experiential learning opportunities, FM educators must consider the context (community) in which students will be practising. The environment should allow them to be active rather than passive participants, exposing them to specific social interactions considered fundamental to experiential learning.[1] Aligned with the social learning theories underpinning experiential learning, the educator can use these sociocultural interactions to influence the outcome of the student's experience.[2]

The FM educator, therefore, must understand the community's cultural practices and beliefs, and show cultural humility. They need to encourage students to understand this phenomenon, through community-based learning activities. For example, sending students with the interprofessional (multidisciplinary) team to visit patients at home. Before, during, and after the visit, students should reflect through identifying their own expectations, observing the patient's environment, and considering how the patient's cultural beliefs may influence their help-seeking behaviours (Chapter 9).

> Cultural humility has the potential to improve relationships and provide opportunities to explore behaviour and health-related beliefs respectfully.

Encouraging students to interact with community care givers/health workers is important as they are often from the community and understand how the health-care system functions. They can play a pivotal role in introducing students to the community culture, and views on their health. These exposures help students understand how the cultural factors at play in the community shape the values, behaviours, and beliefs patients' place on their health needs, and influence clinicians' approaches to diagnosis and treatment. It can be challenging for students to start a conversation with patients about their culture and illness beliefs and tools are available to help. One such tool is the "Exploratory Model Approach".[14] This interview technique helps students understand how the social world affects, and is affected by, illness. It uses six steps to explore the patient's viewpoint of their illness and gain insight into their cultural beliefs[14] (Box 19.2). This provides students with an opening into potentially difficult conversations with patients and helps sensitise them to always consider the patient's cultural background when making decisions on care, whether acute or chronic.

Active participation in learning: Communities of practice

Experiential learning can be summarised as "learning that occurs through reflection on doing"—the two crucial elements being active participation in a learning opportunity and reflection. The student is not the passive recipient of teaching.

BOX 19.2 THE EXPLORATORY MODEL APPROACH[14]

- What do you call this problem?
- What do you believe is the cause of this problem?
- What course do you expect it to take?
- What do you think this problem does inside your body?
- How does it affect your body and your mind?
- What do you most fear about this condition?
- What do you most fear about the treatment?

They must actively participate. In medical education, this often requires consideration of patient safety and organisational compliance. Therefore, the FM educator should not only offer students learning events but observe them while they participate.

> Social interactions with all stakeholders within a clinical learning context are key to active learning.

Lave and Wenger offer theoretical understanding of active participatory learning: "*legitimate peripheral participation*".[15] Learning in a FM environment depends not only on the context (the FM clinic or practice) but also on the social interactions that occur there with healthcare professionals, the educator, the patient, and community members. This participation acknowledges that students need both participation in authentic work-based tasks and supervision to ensure patient safety, within a community of practice. Learning under supervision contributes to the professional identity formation of the future doctor. There are two important components. Students need to participate within the bounds of their own abilities and patient safety. Educators need to observe and supervise the students in order to offer them opportunities that are appropriate for each student's current and next stage of competence.

> Supervised learning ensures patient safety, while enabling the student's professional identity formation.

To nurture student engagement, it helps if students build agentic capacity for self-directed learning before clinical rotations.[16] Five interdependent student capacities have been proposed to enhance student success in clinical environments (Box 19.3). The clinical educator must provide supportive guidance and encourage student participation.

Therefore, to maximise experiential learning, the educator needs to offer students opportunities to participate in authentic work tasks aligned with intended learning outcomes. Progressively more complex roles can be introduced as the student progresses offering greater responsibility. A junior student may do small,

---

BOX 19.3 FIVE WAYS TO ENHANCE STUDENT SELF-DIRECTED LEARNING[16]

- Understanding how to use and extend their learning strategies
- Maximising learning opportunities that are available
- Developing a positive sense of self
- Employing assertive communication
- Developing resilience through mutually supportive peers

deconstructed task components, e.g. taking the blood pressure or examining the chest of a patient presenting with an acute cough. The senior student may participate as a fully-fledged member of the clinical team.

Observing the student enables the educator to decide on the level of supervision each student requires for a particular task, and when they are ready for more complex ones. The FM educator needs to create an encouraging environment in which students are eager to seek and learn from feedback. Feedback on performance helps them to learn, correct mistakes, and, with guidance, reflect on ways to strengthen their performance and prepare for more responsibility. While not all undergraduate curricula have described "Entrustable Professional Activities", the entrustability scale proposed by Chen and colleagues[17] offers an easily understood measure for the progressive supervision of tasks while clearly delineating to the student the required role of the supervisor (Chapter 27). Box 19.4 outlines Chen's entrustable scale.[17]

BOX 19.4 THE ENTRUSTABILITY SCALE[17]

1. *Not allowed* to practise

   ■ Inadequate knowledge/skill (e.g. does not know how to preserve sterile field); not allowed to observe
   ■ Adequate knowledge, some skill; allowed to observe

2. Allowed to practise only under *proactive, full supervision*

   ■ As co-activity with supervisor
   ■ With supervisor in the room; ready to step in as needed

3. Allowed to practise only under *reactive, or on-demand, supervision*

   ■ With supervisor immediately available; all findings double-checked
   ■ With supervisor immediately available; key findings double-checked
   ■ With supervisor distantly available (e.g. by phone); findings reviewed

4. Allowed to practise *unsupervised*

5. Allowed to *supervise others* in practice

Conclusion

This chapter sets out the five consecutive steps the FM educator involved in providing experiential learning opportunities to students should follow:

■ Identify opportunities—students need learning opportunities that enable active participation in authentic clinical tasks to provide the experience on which to reflect.

■ Encourage active student participation.

- Assist reflection—students need assistance to complete the reflective cycle on their experiences to clarify the learning that has happened and define actions for the next learning opportunity.

- Observe the student—structure times to watch the student in action, make decisions on the level of supervision required, and identify the appropriate next opportunities for the student to participate in.

- Construct feedback—offer concrete suggestions on how they might perform even better in future.

References

1. Yardley S, Teunissen PW, Dornan T. Experiential learning: Transforming theory into practice. Med Teach. 2012;34(2):161–4.
2. Yardley S, Teunissen PW, Dornan T. Experiential learning: AMEE Guide no. 63. Med Teach. 2012;34(2):e102–e15.
3. Kolb DA, Boyatzis RE, Mainemelis C. Experiential learning theory: Previous research and new directions. In: Perspectives on thinking, learning, and cognitive styles. Mahwah, NJ: Lawrence Erlbaum Associates; 2001. pp. 193–210.
4. Kolb DA. Experience as the source of learning and development. Upper Saddle River: Prentice Hall; 1984.
5. McLeod S. Kolb's learning styles and experiential learning cycle. Simply Psychol. 2017;5:1–8
6. Mezirow J. (eds.). A transformation theory of adult learning. Adult Education Research Annual Conference Proceedings; 1993: ERIC.
7. Pretorius L, Ford A. Reflection for learning: Teaching reflective practice at the beginning of university study. Int J Learn Teach High Educ. 2016;28(2):241–53.
8. Gibbs G. Learning by doing: A guide to teaching and learning methods. London: Further Education Unit; 2020.
9. Mezirow J. Transformative learning as discourse. J Transform Educ. 2003;1(1):58–63.
10. Artino A, Brydges R, Gruppen LD. Self-regulated learning in healthcare profession education: Theoretical perspectives and research methods. Researching Medical Education. 2015:155–66.
11. Zimmerman BJ. Attaining self-regulation: A social cognitive perspective. In: Handbook of self-regulation. Amsterdam: Elsevier; 2000. p. 13–39.
12. Bandura A. Social foundations of thought and action. Englewood Cliffs, NJ: Prentice Hall; 1986.
13. Clark NM, Zimmerman BJ. A social cognitive view of self-regulated learning about health. Health Educ Behav. 2014;41(5):485–91.
14. Kleinman A, Benson P. Anthropology in the clinic: The problem of cultural competency and how to fix it. PLoS Med. 2006;3(10):e294.
15. Lave J, Wenger E. Situated learning: Legitimate peripheral participation. Cambridge: Cambridge University Press; 1991.
16. Richards J, Sweet L, Billett S. Preparing medical students as agentic learners through enhancing student engagement in clinical education. Asia-Pac J Coop Educ. 2013;14(4):251–63.
17. Chen HC, van den Broek WS, ten Cate O. The case for use of entrustable professional activities in undergraduate medical education. Acad Med. 2015;90(4):431–6.

20

Blended learning

Pramendra Prasad Gupta and Deborah R. Erlich

SUMMARY OF KEY LEARNING POINTS

- Blended learning (BL) combines face-to-face (F2F) education methods with online technology to create an integrated instructional approach.
- Integrating synchronous F2F education with asynchronous online learning is increasingly used in medical schools as it offers more flexible self-directed adult learning.
- Asynchronous online delivery offers students the flexibility to self-direct their learning, improves engagement, and helps students achieve higher and more meaningful learning.
- Family medicine (FM) placements adapt well to BL. Students and tutors are often dispersed geographically across placements, especially in rural settings and some lower- and middle-income countries.
- BL benefits include connectivity, flexibility, self-paced learning, and wider access to expertise.
- Poor technology and digital illiteracy risk inequitable access to learning and student demotivation.
- Research is crucial to ensure BL, post the pandemic, keeps pace with changing patterns in student learning and a rapidly evolving digitally connected world.

Defining blended learning

BL combines F2F education and technology-based learning. It is sometimes called hybrid or mixed mode learning as it integrates elements from the classroom with the digital or virtual world.[1] During technology-based learning processes, students are not required to be physically in one place but may be digitally connected online. Online components can be *synchronous*, where learners and facilitators meet together virtually, such as on videoconferencing platforms, or *asynchronous*, where students

DOI: 10.1201/9781003325734-24

work through resources or assignments at their own pace. Asynchronous learning can be more heavily self-directed.

Alternative definitions exist. Graham defines BL as "systems" that "combine F2F instruction with computer-mediated instruction."[2] Garrison and Kanuka define it as "the thoughtful integration of classroom F2F learning experiences with online learning experiences."[3]

Hege et al.[4] outline several key features of BL upon which this chapter will build:

1. The learners have at least some control over when, where, and how they learn and study.

2. Technology is involved and used to leverage personalisation.

3. Web-based and F2F education are aligned in a meaningful way to offer an integrated learning experience.[4]

> Blended learning combines F2F classroom teaching with online education that students can experience "synchronously" together or "asynchronously" as individuals under self-direction.

What is the difference between "online" and "blended learning"?

Online learning implies 100% online course delivery with few or no F2F sessions.[1] Responsibility for learning primarily rests with the learners. The teacher's role is to guide them. BL combines F2F teaching and the online approach, e.g. 70% online technology and 30% F2F interaction.[5] Students in the BL environment enjoy learning and reviewing at their individual pace but also benefit from interactive F2F sessions.

Types of blended learning

There are three main BL models.[5]

Blended presentation and interaction

Classroom engagement is the primary component of this model. It blends synchronous F2F presentation and interaction with out-of-class, asynchronous online learning exercises. The flipped classroom (or flipped curriculum) approach is a common example increasingly used to replace traditional lectures.[4] A pre-recorded videoed lecture and/or other relevant material is uploaded in advance, enabling students to independently self-direct their learning asynchronously.[6] They then attend a timetabled teacher-facilitated classroom-based session used to field questions, facilitate discussion, and engage learners in deeper understanding of course materials.[1] The opposite can work as well, with in-class events to start, followed by online activities, e.g. discussion forums, online quizzes, and self-assessment.

Blended block

The blended block, or programme flow, model uses sequential "blocks" of F2F learning or online study, often structured to address pedagogical goals or practical constraints, e.g. courses for geographically distributed learners or working professionals with limited opportunities for classroom-based learning.

Fully online

A fully online model may still be considered blended if it incorporates both synchronous learning (e.g. online tutorials) and asynchronous activities (e.g. discussion forums). Table 20.1 summarises and gives examples of the three models.

Various models exist for integrating F2F interactive activities with online learning which are increasingly being used globally by medical schools.

TABLE 20.1 Three models of blended learning

Model 1	Model 2	Model 3
Blended presentation and interaction	**Blended block**	**Fully online**
Activity-focused F2F session(s) blended with online resources	Combination of intensive F2F sessions (one day or longer) and blocks of online learning	Short lecture podcasts combined with online resources and activities
Example	**Example**	**Example**
The flipped curriculum model combines short video lecture podcasts, online resources with F2F tutorials, or seminars for interaction and presentation of group work	A week of intense in-person conference, followed by several weeks or months of home individual study	Weekly online tutorials or seminars for activities and interaction online content and resources

Benefits and challenges of blended learning

The advantages of BL include increased learning skills, greater access to information, improved satisfaction, better learning outcomes, and opportunities to learn with and teach others.[1,7,8] Research has identified the following benefits:

1. *Collaboration at a distance:* Individual students do a task together virtually. Collaboration and community-building from afar suits FM. Students may be assigned singly to practices and distanced from their peers, sometimes across wide geographical spans. Connecting learners in online classrooms is efficient and combats the isolation.

2. *Increased flexibility:* BL enables students to study without time and location barriers but still supported by virtual in-person engagement.[9] Timetabling synchronous teaching in hospitals is easier than in FM where schedules differ

across practices. BL flexibility suits FM rotations. Students can engage in asynchronous teaching as their patient schedules allow.

3. *Increased interaction:* BL offers a platform to facilitate greater interactivity between student peer groups and between students and teachers.

4. *Enhanced learning:* Widening learning formats improves engagement and enables higher, more meaningful learning.[10] The diversity of generalism aligns well with various teaching modalities. Flipping the classroom suits core FM topics. Students can study the basic principles online asynchronously and then spend synchronous classroom time applying the knowledge, solving problems, studying cases, and other higher-level cognitive work.

5. *Increased reach:* Online courses can include student numbers on a far greater scale and offer access to universities, clinics, community health centres, or individual experts with specialist expertise. FM is known for its breadth (Chapter 2). Leveraging BL curricula offers all students access to experts from other institutions in specialist areas, either synchronously via videoconferencing or asynchronously via modules and recorded videos.

6. *Learning to be virtual citizens:* Digital learning introduces new skills. Students can practise projecting themselves socially and academically in an online community of enquiry and master a range of technologies. FM students often follow individual rotas. Teaching students to connect digitally in their own time fits beautifully into the FM clerkship.

FM rotations where students are often attached singly in widely dispersed placements lend themselves well to BL, especially in rural or some low- or middle-income medical schools.

Conversely, BL has challenges:

1. *Technological requirements:* Online learning requires hardware, software, appropriate bandwidth internet, and digital skills. Technology tools must be available and user-friendly, with reliable internet access to support learning in a meaningful way. If unavailable, inequities in access to learning emerge. The COVID-19 pandemic highlighted this.[11,12]

2. *Information technology (IT) literacy:* Students and tutors need the knowledge and IT literacy to engage with BL. Preparation for use of technological tools is required. Lack of IT literacy is a significant barrier to access and quality learning and puts learners with poor IT skills at risk.

In Nepal, during the pandemic, most teachers and students lacked sufficient logistical experience and knowledge to conduct or participate in online teaching. Nepal's broadband speed was unable to support online medical education, which frequently requires access to and transmission of large files and audio-visual material. The experience was similar in Bangladesh.[13]

3. *Lack of self-pacing and self-direction:* Online learning requires student independence and self-management. Research suggests some students watch multiple videoed lectures haphazardly in one go rather than following structured study plans for home viewing and attending live sessions. These students perform worse than those who self-pace well.[14]

4. *Suitability to learners:* Preclinical students may prefer online-based education compared to clinical ones. FM students primarily learn directly from patients in the apprenticeship model. This is nearly impossible to replicate online.[15] If students are unprepared, BL can cause significant emotional stress. The abrupt transition to online learning during the pandemic highlighted this and affected students' readiness to learn.[16]

> Benefits of BL include flexibility, collaboration, and access. When designing BL, challenges such as IT literacy, access technology, and student self-direction must be overcome.

Guidelines for designing blended online courses: Ten tips

We offer ten tips for designing BL experiences.

Tip 1: Develop learning outcomes: First, define clear learning outcomes which align with the medical school curriculum in general and focus on how FM can add value. Decide on assessment tools and ensure these align with the intended learning (Chapter 29). Then, decide how to teach the material. The learning outcomes, assessment tools, and teaching methods may differ significantly from traditional classroom delivery.

Tip 2: Decide how best to blend the learning: FM covers a broad range of clinical topics. Some are difficult to replicate online and are best taught F2F, e.g. physical examination or procedural skills. Some are well suited to online teaching. If F2F curricular time is an option, prioritise material critical to classroom delivery versus synchronous or asynchronous online delivery.

> Some topics are better delivered F2F while some lend themselves well to online learning.

Tip 3: Decide between synchronous and asynchronous learning: For a fully online programme, identify material most appropriate for synchronous, teacher-facilitated learning versus asynchronous, student-paced learning. Pure knowledge transfer may suit videos and self-study material. Application, analysis, case study, and small group activities may work best in a real-time facilitated online virtual meeting. FM, due to its breadth and bio–psychosocial modelling, can help expand the school's digital media library on core generalist topics and skills (Chapter 1). These include advanced communication, motivational interviewing, information mastery, social determinants of health, trauma informed care, and equity and inclusion in medicine.

Tip 4: Plan for synchronous learning: A synchronous online session is a novel educational experience which needs careful design. The content and format of previous F2F classes cannot merely transfer online. Use videoconferencing software tools such as the "Chat" feature, recording role plays, or real-time interactive quizzes or polling. Adjust (usually decrease) the length of a session to suit the synchronous online format.

> Create a thoughtful virtual experience anew. Do not attempt to transfer the old classroom teaching to online settings. Carefully plan to use the full range of available software innovatively.

Tip 5: Set clear expectations for pre-session work: In advance, convey to students how and what to prepare for sessions, e.g. flipped classroom assignments, to maximise their experience in class.

Tip 6: Set ground rules for online synchronous classes: Students must understand how to participate during online sessions.[6] Ground rules include arrive on time; enable video; enable audio; be muted unless called on; turn off cell phones; close other windows and computer programmes; participate from a quiet, undistracted area. State whether food and drink are allowed. Communicate whether you expect questions during or at the session end and how to ask them. Announce the schedule and planned breaks in advance.

Tip 7: Rehearse the technology for synchronous sessions: Arrange real-time technical support or a co-facilitator to help troubleshoot or monitor the Chat feature.

Tip 8: Create active learning opportunities for asynchronous learning: Avoid a mere library of lecture videos. Use self-assessment questions or extension activities. Intersperse information presentations with self or teacher assessments to ensure students get feedback as they progress. Keep all self-study materials, including videos, short, concise, and organised.

Tip 9: Begin and end on time: This applies to all synchronous online education.

Tip 10: Take home messages: Whether F2F is delivered, synchronously in a videoconference, or asynchronously online, conclude with key learning points for participants to take home.

> As in classroom teaching, BL requires setting clear expectations of students and using instructional design principles that engage the learners and enhance retention.

Blending learning as we emerge from COVID-19

Even before the pandemic, student attendance in classroom-based education was declining in favour of at-home studying and asynchronous use of online materials.[16] During the pandemic, a global explosion of BL in various formats occurred as traditional F2F teaching transitioned abruptly to online. Despite the chaos caused by

COVID-19, as we emerge, valuable lessons are being learnt. Lower- and middle-income countries faced unique challenges as highlighted above.[11–13] Globally, early research is revealing mixed responses from students, some valuing self-directed online knowledge learning while some, having experienced technical difficulties, favour a return to the classroom for laboratory and clinical skills teaching.[17,18] Ongoing research is essential to explore how the greater flexibility and benefits of BL can be used strategically for the future.

Conclusion

Technology is rapidly advancing, students' learning styles are changing, and, accelerated by the pandemic, teaching methods are rapidly evolving to keep pace with a digitally connected world. BL is critical to future medical school curricula in nearly all settings. The advantages of scale, access to contributions from non-local experts, and convenience of learning from home can add value to classroom-based courses. FM is especially conducive to BL curricula due to geographically dispersed placements, the breadth of material, and the inclusion of core generalist skills and topics applicable to all medical students entering diverse professions. Many solutions enacted during the pandemic as a response to limitations on group gatherings have been perceived as positive changes to FM education and are likely to persist.[19] Thoughtful planning by course directors can achieve outstanding learning experiences by leveraging the advantages of the classroom with the benefits of virtual connection online.

References

1. Cleveland-Innes M, Wilton D. Guide to blended learning. 2018. Available from: http://oasis.col.org/bitstream/handle/11599/3095/2018_Cleveland-InnesWilton_Guide-to-Blended-Learning.pdf?sequence=1&isAllowed=y
2. Graham CR. Blended learning systems: Definition, current trends and future directions. In: Bonk CJ, Graham CR (eds.), The handbook of blended learning: Global perspectives, local designs. San Francisco: Pfeiffer; 2006. pp. 3–21.
3. Garrison DR, Kanuka H. Blended learning: Uncovering its transformative potential in higher education. Internet High Educ. 2004;7:95–105.
4. Hege I, Tolks D, Adler M, Härtl A. Blended learning: Ten tips on how to implement it into a curriculum in healthcare education. GMS J Med Educ 2020;37(5):Doc45.
5. Northern Illinois University Center for Innovative Teaching and Learning. Blended and distance learning. Instructional guide for university faculty and teaching assistants. 2012. Retrieved from: https://www.niu.edu/citl/resources/guides/instructional-guide
6. Ellaway R, Masters K. AMEE Guide 32: e-learning in medical education part 1: learning, teaching and assessment. Med Teach. 2008;20:455–73.
7. Ilic D, Nordin RB, Glasziou P, Tilson JK, Villanueva E. A randomised controlled trial of a blended learning education intervention for teaching evidence-based medicine. BMC Med Educ. 2015;15:39. doi: 10.1186/s12909-015-0321-6.
8. Woltering H. Blended learning positively affects students' satisfaction and the role of the tutor in the problem-based learning process: Results of a mixed-method evaluation. Adv Health Sci Educ. 2009;14(5):725–38.

9. Zayapragassarazan Z, Kumar S. Blended learning in medical education. NTTC Bull. 2012;19(2):4–5.

10. Lewin LO, Singh M, Bateman BL, Glover PB. Improving education in primary care: Development of an online curriculum using the blended learning model. BMC Med Educ. 2009;9:33.

11. Cecilio-Fernandes D, Parisi MCR, Santos TM, Sandars J. The COVID-19 pandemic and the challenge of using technology for medical education in low and middle income countries. MedEdPublish. 2020;9:74.

12. Connolly N, Abdalla ME. Impact of COVID-19 on medical education in different income countries: A scoping review of the literature. Med Educ Online. 2022;27(1):2040192. doi: 10.1080/10872981.2022.2040192

13. Kabir H, Hassan K, Mitra DK. E-learning readiness and perceived stress among the university students of Bangladesh during COVID-19: A countrywide cross-sectional study. Ann Med. 2021;53(1):2305–14.

14. Zureick AH, Burk-Rafel J, Purkiss JA, Hortsch M. The interrupted learner: How distractions during live and video lectures influence learning outcomes. Anat Sci Educ. 2018;11(4):366–76.

15. Sekine M. Effects of COVID-19 on Japanese medical students' knowledge and attitudes toward e-learning in relation to performance on achievement tests. PLoS One. 2022;17(3):e0265356. doi: 10.1371/journal.pone.0265356

16. Everitt JG, Johnson JM, Burr WH. Why your doctor didn't go to class: Student culture, high-stakes testing, and novel coupling configurations in an allopathic medical school. J Health Soc Behav. 2022. doi: 10.1177/00221465221118584

17. Dyrek N, Wikarek A, Niemiec M, Owczarek AJ, Olszanecka-Glinianowic M, Kocelak P. The perception of e-learning during the SARS-CoV-2 pandemic by students of medical universities in Poland: A survey-based study. BMC Med Educ. 2022;22:529. doi: 10.1186/s12909-022-03600-7

18. Gismalla MDA, Mohamed MS, Ibrahim OSO, Elhassan MMA, Mohamed MNE. Medical students' perception towards E-learning during COVID 19 pandemic in a high burden developing country. BMC Med Educ. 2021;21(1):377.

19. Everard KM, Schiel KZ. Changes in family medicine clerkship teaching due to the COVID-19 pandemic. Fam Med. 2021;53(4):282–4. doi: 10.22454/FamMed.2021.583240

21

Clinical reasoning

Simon Gay

SUMMARY OF KEY LEARNING POINTS

- Pick a recognised definition of clinical reasoning that works best in your own healthcare context.
- Assess where each learner is in their development of clinical reasoning before starting to teach.
- Using a variety of clinical reasoning teaching techniques helps keep the learner stimulated and actively thinking about what they are doing.
- If clinical reasoning is to be accurate and useful, it must account for the needs of the individual patient as well as applying the best available medical evidence.
- Good clinical reasoning includes consideration of social, cultural, and environmental factors for both the individual patient and the society they live in.
- Embedding clinical reasoning as a longitudinal curriculum theme provides a coordinated learning architecture in which suitable levels of challenge can be presented to learners in a sensible sequence and at the most appropriate time.

What can family medicine offer the development of clinical reasoning?

Family medicine (FM) is a superb environment in which to nurture the development of clinical reasoning. Specific features which help to do this include the following:

1. *A safe, supportive learning environment:* This necessitates frequent and sequential feedback from an experienced clinician often over a sufficiently prolonged period of time to allow development of a trusted tutor–student relationship.

2. *Multiple ways to observe and interact with patients:* These include (i) *fly-on-the-wall observations of consultations* between the patient and clinician, (ii) *shared consultations*

DOI: 10.1201/9781003325734-25

with the patient shared between the clinician and the learner, (iii) *"parallel" consultations* where the learner reports back to the clinician supervisor after conducting a consultation with the patient on their own, and then both clinician and learner return to the patient to ensure safe completion of the consultation, (iv) *consulting with patients alone* in very specific circumstances where patient safety can already be assured, such as when implications of blood test results need explaining to a patient, the pre-briefed student can consult with the patient alone, and then simply report back to the clinician on how the consultation went.

3. *Lots of patients:* Globally, large numbers of patients consult in FM daily. Such patient availability offers learners the opportunity to engage in many consultations with patients, one after another. With tailored feedback offered between consultations, learners can quickly act on feedback received while the lesson is still fresh in their memory.

4. *Unfiltered presentations:* Whilst patient numbers are important, patient presentations to FM are usually unfiltered, i.e. triage has not been performed and a preconsultation diagnosis has not been determined. This is a key feature of the FM contribution to clinical reasoning development as they offer ideal experiences for learners to develop their illness scripts. Illness scripts are organised knowledge structures that clinicians mobilise in their brain in relevant clinical reasoning situations. Learners must accumulate these illness scripts over time to build and improve their clinical reasoning skills.[1,2]

> The range of undifferentiated patient presentations in FM enables learners to build illness scripts—an important cognitive process for developing clinical reasoning skills.

However, undifferentiated presentations of patients in FM can at first be daunting for learners used to secondary care clinics and textbook descriptions of clinical presentations. Learners, with support, can make the transformative step across this threshold[3] (Chapter 19).

Definitions of clinical reasoning

The published literature offers many definitions of clinical reasoning without reaching a clear consensus. The term diagnostic reasoning is often interchanged with clinical reasoning when, even though related, they are not synonymous. The educational aim of clinical reasoning tuition in this chapter is ...

> ... *to develop the observation, collection and interpretation of clinical information by healthcare students' so that they can thoughtfully and accurately diagnose, treat and manage patients' health needs, whilst considering the differing social, economic and cultural environments of individual patients.*

What to prioritise for each learner?

Every student has different educational needs. Educators need to quickly determine where a learner's stage of development currently is. A useful tool for deciding where and when to start teaching clinical reasoning to a healthcare student is Pangaro's RIME Model,[4] as outlined in Box 21.1.

Until a learner has the clinical history taking and examination skills to accurately gather information from a patient encounter and concisely and accurately report that information to another healthcare professional, introducing any other aspect of clinical reasoning learning is pointless. Once they can consistently perform these "Reporter" functions, they can start to develop their "Interpreter" skills, i.e. use the information they have collected to work out what they think the patient's diagnoses or problems are. Students who can consistently interpret clinical information with a reasonable degree of accuracy are then ready to formulate logical and feasible patient management plans. Wherever the clinical and cultural context permits, it is good to include the patients in the decision-making process too—this is the "Manager" stage. It takes time for learners to move to the "Educator" stage. At this stage, learners usually have sufficient knowledge, experience, and confidence to engage in more self-directed learning, creating their own questions and finding the correct answers themselves. They are then able to educate their patients and may even start to educate their educators.

Work out where the learner is in their clinical reasoning development before trying to help them improve.

BOX 21.1 THE RIME FRAMEWORK FOR STUDENT PROGRESS[4]

R	"Reporter"
I	"Interpreter"
M	"Manager"
E	"Educator"

Application of best evidence

Healthcare professionals need to be familiar with at least some of the best clinical research evidence available on topics pertinent to their clinical practice. Sackett defined evidence-based medicine as ...

... the conscientious, explicit, and judicious use of current best evidence in making decisions about the care of individual patients.[5]

Note the use of the terms "judicious" and "care of individual patients". Evidence should not simply be used in a "one-size-fits-all" unthinking way. It should be carefully built into the clinical reasoning giving consideration to the individual circumstances, characteristics, and other contextual factors relevant to the specific patient. This is particularly important as most clinical research evidence tends to be single disease focused and has been gathered in affluent, Western populations with little attention to ethnic and cultural diversity. The evidence may be less relevant to people with comorbidities or from different geographical and cultural backgrounds.

> To be successful, clinical reasoning should consider the individual patient's circumstances, and their immediate clinical, social, cultural, and environmental contexts.

Clinical reasoning development techniques

There is little evidence to suggest that teaching the processes involved in clinical reasoning helps clinicians become better diagnosticians. In contrast, we know that specific teaching strategies aimed at building knowledge and understanding lead to improvement.

What follows next is simple guidance on techniques educators can use to facilitate clinical reasoning development. Much of this is based on the UK Clinical Reasoning in Medical Education (CReME) consensus statement.[6]

1. *Help learners to build their understanding:* Encourage learners to use basic science and other prior learning to explain patient presentations and then explicitly clarify their thinking about the presentation.

2. *Encourage structured reflection:* Structured reflection uses prompts, questions, or activities to stimulate deeper thought. Students should be encouraged to ask questions of themselves such as "What's the evidence for this?" They need to be challenged to explain which features of their clinical findings support or question the differential diagnoses they have reached.

3. *Deliberate practice:* It can take approximately 10,000 hours to become expert across a range of skills, e.g. playing the violin or shooting an arrow from a bow. One key process, when moving from novice to expert, is to undertake appropriate, strategic, focused, and goal-orientated activities to improve performance.[7] This is known as "deliberate practice".

    For this to occur, a learner must concentrate fully on the activity itself before receiving and analysing constructive tutor feedback. They must then repeat the same activity. Deliberate practice refines the skill and moves the learner beyond their original performance level.

In clinical reasoning terms, the learner should practise with lots of different cases across as many contexts as possible, and be offered guidance, challenge, and support on their reasoning during each encounter. Real patients with real problems offer students excellent opportunities to learn clinical reasoning, especially in FM if the cases remain undifferentiated and have not yet been filtered into diagnostic subsets. Written and verbal case discussions can also be useful. When developing case-based material, it is important to include from the outset all the information novice healthcare professionals need to address the scenario. This reduces the learner's cognitive load and permits better illness script formation.

> Students in FM must interact with many different patient presentations and contexts, reflecting and acting on feedback to progressively develop their clinical reasoning.

Encourage strategies that structure knowledge around problem-specific concepts: People who are good at clinical reasoning have organised knowledge in their memory more efficiently than people who are less good at clinical reasoning.[8,9] Better structuring of knowledge helps the clinician to move knowledge from one situation to another. This is useful when the context of the reasoning changes. Whilst the evidence base is currently inconclusive, it appears that tools such as decision trees, concept maps, and case discussions within communities of practice may help learners to better structure their clinical knowledge, especially when combined with discussion, guidance, informational feedback, and instructor scaffolding.[10,11]

Making good use of wider science of learning: Certain educational techniques improve learners' retrieval of knowledge performance: see "The Learning Scientists" resource (link at end of chapter) for more detail.

Contrastive learning: Students can learn by comparing and contrasting features of one clinical diagnosis with another, often similar, diagnosis. This can occur visually; for example, by comparing the salient features of an electrocardiogram (ECG) demonstrating complete heart block with a normal ECG, or during discussion by asking learners to compare two similar diagnoses.

Thoughtful challenge: Early in training, it is useful to minimise the cognitive load learners are placed under by starting with low complexity, low fidelity tasks with high instructional support before moving to high complexity, and high fidelity tasks in later years. This is less threatening to learners and makes more of their brainpower available to master the initial stages before moving onto more difficult challenges. The ultimate goal is for students to contribute to the work of the clinical team under appropriate supervision. Feeling useful is a powerful catalyst to learner development. Thoughtful challenge is extremely important and can be extrapolated into the architecture of an entire clinical reasoning–focused curriculum. A good example of this is the recently developed and implemented curriculum at the University of Manchester School of Medical Sciences, UK.[12]

> Enabling students, as their clinical reasoning progresses, to feel appropriately supported and part of the clinical team is a great motivation for learning.

Murtagh's strategy: Once a student has gathered sufficient clinical information, they should be able to offer differential diagnoses. Rather than simply deliver a list of conditions rote learned from a textbook, Murtagh's strategy[13] cognitively "forces" the learner to stratify differential diagnoses into "most likely", "less likely", and must not miss diagnoses they "need to exclude". In addition to demonstrating active clinical reasoning when delivering the differential diagnoses, Murtagh's strategy offers the student a starting point to prioritise what to do next.

SBAR: SBAR[14] is primarily a communication tool commonly used in healthcare environments for patient care handover from one healthcare professional to another (Box 21.2). SBAR is a form of cognitive forcing strategy[15] used to promote healthcare students' clinical reasoning in real time. When presenting their appraisal of clinical situations using SBAR, it is not simply enough to know the clinical findings, the student has to use them to actively inform their assessment and recommendation.

BOX 21.2 SBAR COMMUNICATION TOOL

S	Situation
B	Background
A	Assessment
R	Recommendation

Anchoring to the patient: Healthcare students are good at responding to questions with details learnt from textbooks and other learning materials. However, whilst core knowledge is important, simply regurgitating facts is not enough. Students must be able to apply their learning to the specific context of the patient being cared for. Introducing words when questioning, such as "in this specific patient", anchors the student's thinking to the patient in front of them. It is a good way to check if students have learnt in a logical and patient-centred way.

Tutors must offer constructive feedback using strategies and questions to ensure students have tailored their clinical reasoning answer to the context of the patient facing them.

How to help learners who are struggling with clinical reasoning: Helping learners who are struggling with clinical reasoning despite organised tuition using the above guidance is beyond the scope of this chapter. Tutors seeking more guidance for struggling students are sign-posted to two documents focused on diagnosing and managing clinical reasoning difficulties.[16,17]

Conclusion

Clinical reasoning is a core feature of every practising clinician's working day. For many reasons, FM is well placed to support the development of clinical reasoning. However, providing the appropriate support requires thoughtful planning if FM is to help healthcare learners achieve their full clinical reasoning potential.

Acknowledgements

The author wishes to acknowledge the significant constructive contributions made to this chapter's development by Dr Keith Waddell, Consultant Ophthalmologist at Ruharo Eye Centre and Visiting Professor at the Department of Ophthalmology, Mbarara University Medical School, Uganda. Thank you for challenging my thinking, Keith.

References

1. Feltovich PJ, Barrows HS. Issues of generality in medical problem solving. In: Schmidt HG, De Volder ML. (eds.), Tutorials in problem-based learning: A new direction in teaching the health professions. Vol. 128. Assen: Van Gorcum; 1984. p. 42.
2. Charlin B, Boshuizen HP, Custers EJ, Feltovich PJ. Scripts and clinical reasoning. Med Educ. 2007;41(12):1178–84. doi: 10.1111/j.1365-2923.2007.02924.x.
3. Neve H. Learning to become a primary care professional: Insights from threshold concept theory. Educ Prim Care. 2019;30(1):5–8. doi: 10.1080/14739879.2018.1533390
4. Pangaro L. A new vocabulary and other innovations for improving descriptive in-training evaluations. Acad Med. 1999;74(11):1203–7. doi: 10.1097/00001888-199911000-00012
5. Sackett DL, Rosenberg WMC, Gray JAM, Haynes RB, Richardson WS. Evidence based medicine: What it is and what it isn't. BMJ. 1996;312(7023):71. doi: 10.1136/bmj.312.7023.71
6. Cooper N, Bartlett M, Gay S, Hammond A, Lillicrap M, Matthan J. et al. Consensus statement on the content of clinical reasoning curricula in undergraduate medical education. Med Teach. 2021; 43(2):152–59. doi: 10.1080/0142159X.2020.1842343
7. Ericsson K, Krampe R, Tesch-Römer C. The role of deliberate practice in the acquisition of expert performance. Psychol Rev. 1993;100(3):363–406. doi: 10.1037//0033-295X.100.3.363
8. Bordage G, Lemieux M. Structuralism and medical problem solving. Int Semiotic Spect. 1987;7(1):3–4.
9. Grant J, Marsden P. The structure of memorized knowledge in students and clinicians: An explanation for diagnostic expertise. Med Educ. 1987;21(2):92–98. doi: 10.1111/j.1365-2923.1987.tb00672.x.
10. Choudhari SG, Gaidhane AM, Desai P, Srivastava T, Mishra V, Zahiruddin SQ. Applying visual mapping techniques to promote learning in community-based medical education activities. BMC Med Educ. 2021;21(1):1–4. doi: 10.1186/s12909-021-02646-3
11. Pudelko B, Young M, Vincent-Lamarre P, Charlin B. Mapping as a learning strategy in health professions education: A critical analysis. Med Educ. 2012;46(12):1215–25. doi: 10.1111/medu.12032
12. Singh M, Collins L, Farrington R, et al. From principles to practice: Embedding clinical reasoning as a longitudinal curriculum theme in a medical school programme. Diagnosis (Berl). 2021;9(2):184–94. doi: 10.1515/dx-2021-0031

13. Murtagh J. Common problems: A safe diagnostic strategy. Aust Fam Physician. 1990;19(5):733–34.
14. SBAR Tool: Situation-Background-Assessment-Recommendation. IHI—Institute for Healthcare Improvement [Internet]. Ihi.org. 2022 (Accessed 11 March 2022). Available from: http://www.ihi.org/resources/Pages/Tools/SBARToolkit.aspx
15. Croskerry P. Cognitive forcing strategies in clinical decision making. Ann Emerg Med. 2003;41(1):110–20. doi: 10.1067/mem.2003.22
16. Audétat MC, Laurin S, Dory V, Charlin B, Nendaz MR. Diagnosis and management of clinical reasoning difficulties: Part I. Clinical reasoning supervision and educational diagnosis. Med Teach. 2017;39(8):792–6. doi: 10.1080/0142159X.2017.1331033
17. Audétat MC, Laurin S, Dory V, Charlin B, Nendaz MR. Diagnosis and management of clinical reasoning difficulties: Part II. Clinical reasoning difficulties: Management and remediation strategies. Med Teach. 2017;39(8):797–801. doi: 10.1080/0142159X.2017.1331034

Other resources

- UK Clinical Reasoning in Medical Education. Available from: https://creme.org.uk/index.html

- The Learning Scientists. Available from: https://www.learningscientists.org/downloadable-materials

- Society to Improve Diagnosis in Medicine. Available from: https://www.improvediagnosis.org/

22

Communication skills

Mora Claramita and Jillian Benson

SUMMARY OF KEY LEARNING POINTS

- All medical students should learn patient-centred communication skills to ensure accurate diagnosis and management, collaborative healthcare services, and effective health outcomes.
- Undergraduates need communication skills contextualised within an understanding of diversity to fully support patients' perspectives of their culture, gender, social status, or age.
- A simple framework, "greet–invite–discuss", enables students to learn culturally adaptable patient-centred communication skills to achieve shared management decisions.
- Complex health problems in FM need strategic, flexible communication to build relationships between family doctors, patients, families, community, and other health professionals.
- FM educators are well placed to introduce undergraduates to additional generalist skills: motivational interviewing, shared decision-making, and dealing with uncertainty.
- Establishing strong therapeutic relationships with patients to ensure compliance with medication is crucial. Guiding students using frameworks for doing this is important.

Introduction

Eighty percent of a diagnosis can be established during the history-taking phase of the doctor–patient consultation.[1] This principle applies only if a patient-centred communication style is used. Patient-centred care can be defined as "providing care that is respectful of, and responsive to, individual patient preferences, needs, and values". It must ensure that patient values guide all clinical decisions.[2] Doctors facilitate a two-way conversation to allow patients to express their concerns and priorities.[3]

DOI: 10.1201/9781003325734-26

The structure of the patient-centred communication style: The greet–invite–discuss

There are many guidelines on how to approach patient-centred communication. In this section, an easy-to-use framework is introduced, based on international guidance but more sensitive to cultural differences.[4,5] There are three stages: "greet–invite–discuss".

The "greet" stage

The "greet" stage can affect the overall consultation. The doctor's readiness for the consultation is evidenced by an allocated patient appointment time, well-prepared medical records, as few interruptions as possible, and communication aides such as an interpreter, if necessary. Good rapport is essential to put the patient at ease to share their story. Patients from more hierarchical cultures, e.g. Asian or African, may be familiar with (but not necessarily accept) a social gap between people and a one-way, more doctor-centred style.[5,6] In Western countries, e.g. Europe or North America, relationships tend more towards partnerships (Chapter 12). With increasing global migration, cross-cultural communication skills have become essential throughout the world.

> The undergraduate curriculum must prepare future doctors for global migration and the need for a culturally sensitive and flexible approach to patient-centred communication.

The "invite" stage of the consultation

The patient as an expert

It is important that students respect the patient as an expert. They need to learn how to open a consultation by asking a series of open-ended questions, as outlined in Box 22.1. Any additional questions should aim to probe deeper into the stories in a more focused manner, e.g. "Please tell me more about it?"

Arthur Kleinman proposed eight questions, summarised in Box 22.2, to explore the patient's perspective on their problems. These questions should be expanded depending on the patient's answers until a deep understanding of the patient's beliefs, fears, perceptions, and expectations is gained.[7]

BOX 22.1 OPEN QUESTIONS

- How are you doing today?
- How do you feel?
- What can I do for you?
- Tell me about what matters to you?

> ### BOX 22.2 KLEINMAN'S EIGHT QUESTIONS[7]
>
> 1. What do you call your problem? What name do you give it?
> 2. What do you think has caused it?
> 3. Why did it start when it did?
> 4. What does your sickness do to your body? How does it work inside you?
> 5. How severe is it? Will it get better soon or take longer?
> 6. What do you fear most about your sickness?
> 7. What are the chief problems your sickness has caused for you (personally, family, work, etc.)?
> 8. What kind of treatment do you think you should receive? What are the most important results you hope to receive from the treatment?

The doctor as expert

Once the patient's ideas, concerns, and expectations are clear, students can move to ask closed questions, potentially open to an answer of either "yes" or "no", centred on what is happening clinically. The fundamentals of history-taking can be followed asking "when", "where", "current/past/family history", "duration", "aggravating factors", "relieving factors", etc.[1,4] The student can then follow with a medical explanation of what the symptoms mean, differential diagnoses, and any uncertainties. Subsequently, the patient can begin to follow the student's clinical reasoning (Chapter 21) and ask questions or add more information. Shared thinking between doctor and patient can achieve a more accurate diagnosis and deliverable management plan. Ultimately, the student should learn to summarise the consultation and discuss the investigations needed.

> Students must learn how to use open questions and respect the patient's agenda before moving to closed questions to build on the doctor's agenda of clinical reasoning.

The "discuss" stage

This is the "informed and shared decision-making stage".[8] Steps of "choice, options, and decision" assist the doctor and patient to conduct a two-way conversation and reach a management plan acceptable to both. Students should be encouraged to use decision support tools, i.e. illustrations, pictures, or visual aids, that help patients understand and reach decisions, e.g. why a treatment is more effective or making a choice between lifestyle or medication. These illustrations can assist doctors, patients, and their families to explore their initial preferences and deliberate on the pros and cons of each option.

For patients from more hierarchical cultures, shared discussion with their doctor may be unfamiliar. They might respond with "yes, doctor", not necessarily as an agreement, but more a polite response to an instruction from someone from a perceived higher status.[5] Therefore, students should learn to become aware of any hesitation by patients, and acknowledge, explore, and discuss any social gap carefully. Cultures with more hierarchical structures may have a more collectivist approach to decision-making involving family members, relatives, or community members[5] (Chapter 12). The best health outcomes will only be achieved with full patient understanding and consent to any clinical decisions or management. The holistic generalist approach fundamental to primary care (Chapter 1) offers an ideal context for FM doctors to role model the shared management achievable through patient-centred communication.

> Observing FM doctors at work in the holistic generalist context enables students to learn the importance of achieving shared decision-making with patients.

The therapeutic relationship

A high proportion of patients presenting to family practitioners suffer from psychological disorders, often experiencing long-term consequences for themselves and their families but remaining undiagnosed. Due to the fear of stigma, such patients may prefer to be cared for by their FM doctor, despite the availability of other health professionals and mental health organisations.[9] A strong therapeutic relationship is essential in all FM consultations to achieve patient satisfaction, save time, and increase compliance with prescribed medication.[10]

Many scales have been developed to quantify a high-quality FM–patient relationship. These do not really measure the quality of the relationship but can offer some important insights into the level of therapeutic alliance.[11] The ratings offer a basis for reflection and discussion on aligning the doctor's agenda of "friendship, respect, commitment, affirmation, recognition, responsiveness, positive regard, empathy, trust, and receptivity, with the patient's lifeworld, honesty, and reflexivity. This provides an ongoing focus on care to embrace prevention, illness management, and rehabilitation".[12]

> The ongoing relationship between patients and FM doctors builds shared understanding and a therapeutic alliance to improve compliance and, ultimately, healthcare outcomes.

FM consultations are often complex. Many barriers need to be addressed. The therapeutic relationship can be influenced by "doctor" issues, e.g. communication style, cultural awareness, ethnocentrism, and adhering to evidence inappropriate to the context. In addition, "patient" issues, either conscious or unconscious, can influence the interaction, e.g. health literacy; social media; family, spiritual, or cultural beliefs; and comorbidities. Organisational and sociopolitical issues can affect the ability of the doctor and the patient to communicate freely. These include time pressure, lack of collaborative teamwork, poverty, inadequate health infrastructure, political turmoil, and institutional racism.[13]

Multimorbidity

Many patients seen by family doctors have several chronic diseases. This makes delivery of care not only more clinically complex, but also involves frequent consultations, multiple medications, and requires liaison with the wider health system. Developing management plans that involve lifestyle changes, compliance with medication regimes, and coordination of the allied health team must be delivered in a patient- and family-centred manner (Chapter 9).

By observing FM doctors at work, students can learn how to build strong partnerships, which balance patient and doctor priorities, and prove more successful than just giving advice. Motivational interviewing has expanded beyond its original use of addressing addictive behaviour, to be embraced by all spheres of medicine. Learning this skill offers students a way of understanding and facilitating behaviour change and improving a patient's motivation to work with the FM team to decrease their risks and improve their health.[14]

A model of "engaging, focusing, evoking and planning" can help explore options, as patients with multimorbidity often feel overwhelmed by all the management issues. An "importance" and "confidence" scale can be coupled with reflection to shift the focus away from topics that are unhelpful or causing discord. The scale could be as simple as, for example, "using a scale from 1 to 10 (from the least to the highest), how do you rate your confidence to leave the house; both before and after taking the medicine?" This kind of question will help patients and doctors to understand how the illness can change with medication and/or lifestyle changes.

"Evoking" is about listening for the patient's beliefs, preferences, strengths and values, and building on their positive "change talk".[14] The shared plan achieved in this way will be coupled with eliciting the patient's knowledge about the management options and confirming that they understand and accept the agreed approach.

Uncertainty

Uncertainty is a hallmark of FM practice (Chapter 24). Primary care offers a good context for students to begin to come to terms with this aspect of medicine. Doctors can never be sure of the outcome. However, disclosure and discussion of the uncertainty inherent in many medical decisions are essential for true shared decision-making and patient-centred care.[15] Communicating the uncertainty inherent in any management plan, and the subsequent safety-netting that should ensue to manage risk and known or unknown adverse outcomes, is often neglected. Students must be introduced to the challenges of communicating uncertainty which include doctor issues such as fear, feelings of vulnerability, cultural issues, time, and personality. Patients may not wish, or have the numerical or psychological capacity, to hear about uncertainties.

> Many consultations in FM involve undifferentiated presentations and enable students to experience how to communicate uncertainty and balance risk with patients.

The cultural influence within the FM context

One main issue in FM is the influence of culture on health outcomes. The story below centres on one country but can be utilised to reflect and learn about global differences between patients' and doctors' perceptions when approaching health outcomes.

THE STORY OF THE SUKRI FAMILY

Mr. Sukri is a farmer with a schoolteacher wife and two young daughters. He presents with a cough. They live in a small house with a soil floor, a toilet built by student volunteers, and beds of bamboo. He has been diagnosed with pulmonary tuberculosis (TB) and given a free six-month course of treatment from the nearest primary care clinic (Puskesmas). After six months, he has not responded to treatment. The doctor was confused as he felt Mr. Sukri had received all the necessary information. The Puskesmas healthcare team had followed the full protocol—of education, close contact screening, health promotion for the village people, and training Mrs. Sukri to be the drug-observer advocate.

The illustration is typical of many doctor–patient consultations globally. Reflecting on this real-life scenario with students can open their eyes to the complexity of patient management, how to check patient understanding, and achieve active compliance with treatment. A patient with a cough may not expect a serious diagnosis and think he has something less sinister. The doctor has correctly diagnosed TB. If patients do not fully comprehend, management is less likely to be successful. Curiosity and exploration of the patients' perceptions can be highly challenging for medical students. It requires deep listening, reflective observations, and an ability to step back to assess the situation.[4,5]

> Learning reflective practice underpins the patient-centred communication skills needed to establish a strong therapeutic relationship and achieve patient compliance.

Various frameworks exist to help students learn to listen deeply when they are gathering information and then explain and plan management comprehensively addressing patients' cultural beliefs and social background. The Calgary Cambridge framework[16] (Figure 22.1) emphasises to students the need to follow the structure of traditional

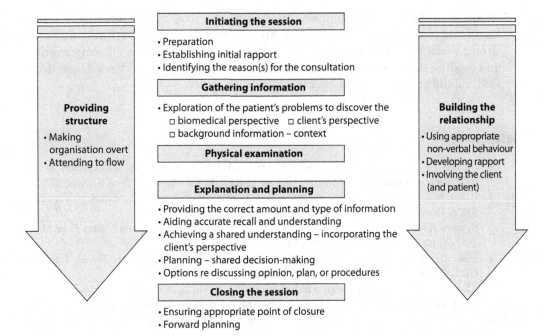

Initiating the session

- Preparation
- Establishing initial rapport
- Identifying the reason(s) for the consultation

Gathering information

- Exploration of the patient's problems to discover the
  □ biomedical perspective   □ client's perspective
  □ background information – context

Physical examination

Explanation and planning

- Providing the correct amount and type of information
- Aiding accurate recall and understanding
- Achieving a shared understanding – incorporating the
  client's perspective
- Planning – shared decision-making
- Options re discussing opinion, plan, or procedures

Closing the session

- Ensuring appropriate point of closure
- Forward planning

Providing structure

- Making organisation overt
- Attending to flow

Building the relationship

- Using appropriate non-verbal behaviour
- Developing rapport
- Involving the client (and patient)

FIGURE 22.1 The Calgary Cambridge framework.[16]

history-taking, as learnt in secondary care, and simultaneously build a relationship with the patient; a skill which can be effectively learnt in FM where the approach is more holistic. Alternatively Neighbour offers five checkpoints: "connecting", "summarising", "handing over", "safety netting", and "housekeeping"[17] which students can find useful in learning to handle uncertainty (Chapter 24). Supporting students to summarise back to the patient what they have heard when data gathering, and before moving on, is a useful technique to check that they have listened effectively.

Informed and shared decision-making are the most complex and time-consuming part of a consultation. A gap from the beginning between the patient's and the doctor's perceptions and understanding can affect the final health outcome.

In our example, the first two months of TB treatment can be difficult because of medication side effects. Mrs. Sukri has to become the patient's advocate, and provide full psychosocial, and even financial, support, as she substitutes as the family breadwinner. Unless the therapeutic relationship is strong, they may decide to discontinue the medication instead of asking questions about alternative treatments. This is a community problem as well as a personal problem. Tuberculosis is a good example of how lack of effective patient-centred communication for health concerns can impact on health outcomes in the wider community.

Conclusion

Patient-centred communication and shared decision-making are fundamental skills family doctors can role model for medical students. FM provides an excellent context for students to learn the skills needed to develop strong patient-centred relationships by understanding the patient's perspective, using culturally sensitive communication skills and dealing with uncertainty through self-reflection. A strong therapeutic collaboration built on exploration of various choices, assisting and guiding the patient to make an informed, confident, and evidence-based decision, should ensure the most effective health outcomes.

References

1. Bickley LS, Szilagyl PG, Hoffman RM, Soriano RP (eds.). Chapters 1 and 2, Bates' guide to physical examination and history taking. 13th ed. Philadelphia: Wolters Kluwer; 2001.
2. Baker A. Crossing the quality chasm: A new health system for the 21st century (Vol. 323, 7322). British Medical Journal Publishing Group; 2001. p. 1192.
3. Epstein RM, Street RL. The values and value of patient-centered care. Ann Fam Med. 2011;9(2):100–03. doi: 10.1370/afm.1239
4. Silverman J, Kurtz S, Draper J. Skills for communicating with patients. 3rd ed. London: CRC Press; 2016. doi: 10.1201/9781910227268
5. Claramita M, Susilo AP. Improving communication skills in the Southeast Asian health care context. Perspect Med Educ. 2014;3(6):474–9. doi: 10.1007/s40037-014-0121-4
6. Hofstede G. Dimensionalizing cultures: The Hofstede model in context. Online Read Psychol Culture. 2011;2(1). doi: 10.9707/2307-0919.1014
7. Kleinman A. The illness narratives: Suffering, healing, and the human condition. New York: Basic Books; 1988.
8. Elwyn G, Frosch D, Thomson R, Joseph-Williams N, Lloyd A, Kinnersley P, Cording E, Tomson D, Dodd C, Rollnick S, Edwards A, Barry M. Shared decision making: A model for clinical practice. J Gen Intern Med. 2012;27(10):1361–67. doi: 10.1007/s11606-012-2077-6
9. Ardito RB, Rabellino D. Therapeutic alliance and outcome of psychotherapy: Historical excursus, measurements, and prospects for research. Front Psychol. 2011;2:270. doi: 10.3389/fpsyg.2011.00270
10. King's Fund. Improving the quality of care in general practice. Report of an independent inquiry commissioned by the King's Fund. London: The King's Fund; 2011.
11. Greenhalgh T, Heath I. Measuring quality in the therapeutic relationship: Part 1: Objective approaches. Qual Saf Health Care. 2010;19(6):475–78. doi: 10.1136/qshc.2010.043364.
12. Greenhalgh T, Heath I. Measuring quality in the therapeutic relationship: Part 2: Subjective approaches. Qual Saf Health Care. 2010;19(6):479–83. doi: 10.1136/qshc.2010.043372.
13. Benson J. Concordance: An alternative term to 'compliance' in the Aboriginal population. Aust Fam Physician. 2005;34(10):831–5.
14. McKenzie KJ, Pierce D, Gunn JM. Guiding patients through complexity: Motivational interviewing for patients with multimorbidity. Aust J Gen Pract. 2018;47(1/2):8–13.
15. Simpkin AL, Armstrong KA. Communicating uncertainty: A narrative review and framework for future research. J Gen Intern Med. 2019;34(11):2586–91. doi: 10.1007/s11606-019-04860-8.
16. Kurtz SM, Silverman JD. The Calgary-Cambridge references observation guides: An aid to defining the curriculum and organising the teaching in communication training programmes. Med Educ. 1996;30:83–9.
17. Neighbour R. The inner consultation: How to develop an effective and intuitive consulting style. 2nd ed. Taylor & Francis; 2015

23

Clinical and procedural skills

Eric Wong and Krishna Suvarnabhumi

SUMMARY OF KEY LEARNING POINTS

- Clinical skills are discrete and observable acts of patient care that include proficiency in communication, physical examination, treatment/therapeutics, and practical procedures.
- Medical students must graduate with the clinical skills needed to meet the health needs of populations they will serve as postgraduate trainees or independent practitioners.
- It is important students learn the skills to work efficiently and accurately to resolve problems (routine expertise) and to navigate and solve new problems (adaptive expertise).
- The generalist, community context of family medicine (FM), offers an ideal environment to teach, assess, and give formative feedback on students' clinical skills development.
- When teaching clinical and procedural skills, it is important to include the declarative and procedural knowledge and the clinical reasoning associated with the skill being learnt.
- Clinical skills are not innate and must be learnt in explicit steps moving from demonstration to simulation to supervised performance on patients. Practice is essential.
- Formative assessment, giving students constructive feedback on learning, and summative methods, confirming achievement of appropriate competency standards, are crucial.

What are clinical and procedural skills?

When designing the medical school curriculum, to ensure that medical students on graduation can adequately and safely meet societal needs, a clear understanding is essential of what clinical and procedural skills to include or exclude and in what context they are best learnt. FM provides an excellent environment for teaching and assessing many of these skills which lie in the generalist domain.

DOI: 10.1201/9781003325734-27

There is a lack of consensus on the definition of clinical skills in the medical community.[1] Consequently, there is no agreement on how best to teach clinical and procedural skills. Michels et al.[1] used a Delphi consensus methodology with 26 UK medical educationalists to address this gap. They concluded that clinical skills comprised domains of physical examination, communication, treatment/therapeutic skills, and practical procedures with, or without, integration across these domains. This is consistent with the Association of American Medical Colleges who define a clinical skill as "any discrete and observable act of medical care".[2] The Accreditation Council for Graduate Medical Education (ACGME) states, under the domain of patient care, that all medical residents are expected to demonstrate competence in the areas outlined in Box 23.1.[3]

It is helpful to define the limits of what we mean by procedural skills. The Council of Academic FM Consensus Statement for Procedural Training in FM Residency use this definition: "The mental and motor activities required to execute a manual task involving patient care".[4] This essentially limits procedures to manual tasks that have both a technical component and interpretation component. It excludes procedures that involve only interpretation, e.g. interpretation of an electrocardiogram or primarily clinical decision-making.

> Because there is no consensus for the definition of a clinical skill, it is critical in curriculum development to first define it.

Given that Chapters 21 and 22 address clinical reasoning and communication skills, we will focus our discussion on physical examination skills and procedural skills.

Why teach clinical and procedural skills?

This important question impacts on how to teach clinical and procedural skills in FM. It sets out a philosophical approach to training in this area.

The ultimate aim is for medical schools to be socially accountable and meet the population's health needs (Chapters 3 and 8). The World Health Organisation (WHO)

BOX 23.1 ACCREDITATION COUNCIL FOR GRADUATE MEDICAL EDUCATION (ACGME) CORE CLINICAL SKILLS COMPETENCIES REQUIRED FOR PATIENT CARE[3]

- Gather essential and accurate information about the patient.
- Counsel patients and family members.
- Make informed diagnostic and therapeutic decisions.
- Prescribe and perform essential medical procedures.
- Provide effective health management, maintenance, and prevention guidance.

defines this as "the obligation to direct their education, research and service activities towards addressing the priority health concerns of the community, region, and/or nation they have a mandate to serve".[5] The end goal is to ensure that medical school graduates have the clinical and procedural skills to adequately and safely address the health requirements of the local population they will be working for, whether in the context of independent practice or postgraduate training. The generalist approach of FM, situated within the local community, provides an ideal environment for learning these skills.

What physical examination skills and procedural skills should we teach?

The role of medical training is to assist practitioners to become master adaptive learners equipped with both routine expertise (the ability to efficiently and accurately resolve problems) and adaptive expertise (the ability to navigate new problems through learning innovative problem-solving).[6] The medical school curriculum must define which physical examination and procedural skills are most important for addressing the population's health needs and which are most likely to assist the development of adaptive expertise.

Other important factors may include the following:

■   Local and regional epidemiology

■   Expectations of medical graduates upon graduation

■   Local and regional resources in the educational and health systems

■   Local and regional health system setup and culture

Once the context and influences are understood, the skills that medical students must perform competently can be refined to prioritise those appropriate to undergraduate training acknowledging that, globally, many graduates then enter a period of supervised residency.

Published work on how to define which physical examination and procedural skills must be taught and assessed is lacking. Common methodologies include consensus approaches such as the nominal group technique and the Delphi method[4,7,8] and, for procedure skills, survey studies.[9] The Council of Academic Family Medicine Consensus Statement for Procedural Training in FM Residency[4] offers a possible approach. It emphasises the importance of involving FM doctors alongside secondary care specialists. It translates well for physical examination skills and includes the following key processes:

■   From the initial resultant, often long, list identify a sublist (A) focusing on the common, simple skills and procedures a medical student *must* competently and safely perform on graduation. It does not need to be exhaustive.

■   Assuming students are competent in performing the prioritised list (A) procedures and agree on a list (B) of procedures, all undergraduate medical graduates should be adequately trained to perform. Generally, competence in these procedures will infer adaptive expertise in procedural skills.

■ A final list (C) will consist of more complex or advanced skills and procedures where training may be offered depending on local needs and practice patterns. Competence is generally not expected for all medical graduates.

A process that includes family physicians' input is critical to the development of an appropriate list of physical examination and procedural skills to be taught in medical schools.

Some countries, e.g. the UK, have a national undergraduate competency-based curriculum (Chapter 10) with clear clinical and procedural skill outcomes against which students are assessed and medical school performance can be regulated.[10] The Association of Faculties of Medicine in Canada has also published a guide that outlines the expected levels of competencies for various clinical and procedural skills for the undergraduate medical student at entry to clerkship and then at the time of graduation.[11] There are some concrete postgraduate examples to help design undergraduate training; for example, (i) the North America Council of Academic FM consensus statement for procedural training in FM residency[4] and the UK clinical examination procedures and skills for postgraduate FM training workplace-based assessment (WPBA).[12] In Australia[13] and South Africa,[14] Delphi studies have built national consensus on the clinical procedural skills outcomes expected of FM training programmes and the South East Asia WHO Regional Office has a recommended set of procedural skills for FM trainees.[15] It is important to recognise that modifications are required to meet each medical school's curriculum, the country's healthcare context, and the level of competency expected of medical students as they progress through the course.

Family physicians resource a defined community.[16] FM is best positioned to contribute to medical schools' efforts in determining the population's health needs and to prioritise what clinical and procedural skills to teach. This is especially true in a situation where medical graduates may start work independently in the community upon medical school graduation.

How to teach physical examination skills and procedural skills?

There is no consensus on how best to teach physical examination and procedural skills. Michels et al.[1] state it is important to include declarative knowledge (e.g. underlying anatomy and physiology), procedural knowledge (how to perform the skill), and clinical reasoning (e.g. diagnostic, and clinical decision-making) clearly identifying which domains are being taught. Different underlying educational principles and theories may influence which approach to take. Burgess et al.[17] confirm this, emphasising that "becoming competent in a skill involves three main components: knowledge, communication and performance". They offer some specific tips as outlined in Box 23.2.

The teaching of physical examination and procedural skills is more than just teaching the performance of the motor tasks. The cognitive aspects of the skills must also be taught.

> ### BOX 23.2 SPECIFIC TIPS FOR TEACHING CLINICAL SKILLS AND PROCEDURES[15]
>
> - *Include the fundamentals:* e.g. handwashing.
> - *Demonstration:* Provide clear demonstrations for learners to see.
> - *Integrate theory with practice:* If learners see the evidence behind the action, this promotes clinical reasoning.
> - *Break skills/procedures down into steps:* Find out what the learners already know, and proceed from there.
> - *Use collaborative problem-solving:* Allow learners to work together towards a solution.
> - *Provide feedback:* That is clear and constructive, in an appropriate environment

Burgess et al.[17] and Garcia-Rodriguez [18] recommend a six-step approach developed by Sawyer et al.[19] for procedural skill acquisition and maintenance:

1. *Learn:* Knowledge acquisition.
2. *See:* Observation of the procedure.
3. *Practice:* Deliberate practice using simulation.
4. *Prove:* Competency is assessed.
5. *Do:* The procedure is performed on a patient, with direct supervision until the learner is entrusted to perform the procedure independently.
6. *Maintain:* Continued clinical practice, supplemented by simulation-based training.

Finally, Burgess et al.[17] highlight the importance of simulation-based training in the acquisition of procedural skills for deliberate practice and skills maintenance. Other authors offer more economical ways of using simulation for procedural skills training.[19–21]

> Clinical skills are not innate. Break the learning into explicit steps. Move from demonstration to simulation to supervised performance on patients. Emphasise practice is essential to improve.

How to assess physical examination skills and procedural skills?

We briefly highlight important principles for clinical skills assessment. Chapter 27 on the assessment of clinical competency and Chapter 29 on assessment tools offer full detail. There are two major components of procedural skills assessment, almost certainly transferable to physical examination skills.[4,22] Firstly, the assessment of discreet individual procedural skills. Secondly, the assessment of the adaptive expertise.

Individual procedural skills are usually assessed using validated assessment tools (Chapter 29). The assessment of adaptive expertise may predict someone's ability to learn and conduct new procedures to deal with evolving community needs. This requires additional performance data on individual skills.[22] As this approach was designed for postgraduate FM training, medical schools will need to modify them to fit the competence level expected of students according to their position on the course and the environment.

Assessment should be both formative and summative.[15] For a formative approach, trainers must provide regular constructive feedback to trainees to ensure that they set personal goals for improvement. Summative assessments at the end of a training period will need to be constructively aligned with the environment in which trainees learn.[23]

> It is important to encourage students to practise and maintain their skills giving formative constructive feedback to ensure they strive to move beyond competence to excellence

Conclusion

A clear understanding of clinical and procedural skills and the ultimate educational goals are critical before deciding what, when, and how to teach them. Social accountability must be considered to ensure students graduate with the skills needed to address local and regional health system factors and the healthcare needs of the population to be served. Family physicians' input is critical as they hold extensive generalist knowledge of their local communities.

While there is no consensus on how to best teach clinical skills, focus on cognitive and technical aspects is important. Assessment should be *formative* offering constructive personalised feedback and *summative* using tools validated to confirm that competency has been achieved appropriate to the level of training. To address adaptive expertise, performance data is important.

Teaching resources

- Canadian Family Physician video series on procedures: www.cfp.ca/content/by/section/Video%20Series

- MededPortal: https://www.mededportal.org/

- American Family Physician articles on various procedures: https://www.aafp.org/afp/topicModules/viewTopicModule.htm?topicModuleId=87#0

- Medscape Clinical Procedures: https://emedicine.medscape.com/clinical_procedures

References

1. Michels MEJ, Evans DE, Blok GA. What is a clinical skill? Searching for order in chaos through a modified Delphi process. Med Teach. 2012;34(8):e573–e81.
2. Recommendations for Clinical Skills Curricula for Undergraduate Medical Education. Task force on the clinical skills education of medical students. The Association of American Medical Colleges. 2005. Available from: https://store.aamc.org/downloadable/download/sample/sample_id/174/ (Accessed 8 January 2022).
3. Exploring the ACGME Core Competencies: Patient Care and Procedural Skills (Part 3 of 7). Available from: https://knowledgeplus.nejm.org/blog/patient-care-procedural-skills/ (Accessed 8 January 2022).

4. Council of Academic Family Medicine Consensus Statement for Procedural Training in Family Medicine Residency. Available from: https://www.afmrd.org/d/do/966 (Accessed 8 January 2022).

5. Boelen C, Heck JE. Division of Development of Human Resources for Health. Defining and measuring the social accountability of medical schools/Charles Boelen and Jeffery E. Heck. World Health Organization; 1995. Available from: https://apps.who.int/iris/handle/10665/59441 (Accessed 8 January 2022).

6. Cutrer WB, Miller B, Pusic MV, Mejicano G, Mangrulkar RS, Gruppen LD et al. Fostering the development of master adaptive learners: A conceptual model to guide skill acquisition in medical education. Acad Med. 2017;92:70–75.

7. Wetmore SJ, Rivet C, Tepper J, Tatemichi S, Donoff M, Rainsberry P. Defining core procedure skills for Canadian family medicine training. Can Fam Physician. 2005;51(10):1364–5.

8. Association of Faculties of Medicine of Canada. AFMC National Clinical Skills Working Group evidence-based clinical skills document: Introduction. Available from: http://clinicalskills.machealth.ca/index.php/content/intro (Accessed 8 January 2022).

9. Battaglia F, Sayed C, Merlano M, McConnell M, Ramnanan C, Rowe J et al. Identifying essential procedural skills in Canadian undergraduate medical education. Can Med Educ J. 2020;11(6):e17–e23.

10. General Medical Council UK Outcomes for Graduates: Practical skills and procedures. 2018. Available from: https://www.gmc-uk.org/education/standards-guidance-and-curricula/standards-and-outcomes/outcomes-for-graduates (Accessed 31 January 2023).

11. Association of Faculties of Medicine of Canada National Clinical Skills Working Group Evidence-Based Clinical Skills Document. Available from: http://clinicalskills.machealth.ca/index.php/content/intro (Accessed 31 January 2023).

12. Workplace Based Assessment WPBA. Available from: https://www.rcgp.org.uk/training-exams/training/workplace-based-assessment-wpba.aspx (Accessed 10 January 2022).

13. Sylvester S, Magin P, Sweeney K, Morgan S, Henderson K. Procedural skills in general practice vocational training what should be taught? Aust Fam Physician. 2011;40(1/2):50–54.

14. Mash B, Couper I, Hugo J. Building consensus on clinical procedural skills for South Africa family medicine training using the Delphi technique. SA Fam Pract. 2006;48(10):14–14e.

15. World Health Organization. Family medicine report of a regional scientific working group meeting on core curriculum. New Delhi: World Health Organization Regional Office for South-East Asia; 2003.

16. Rosser W. Sustaining the 4 principles of family medicine in Canada. Can Fam Physician. 2006;52(10):1191–2, 1196–7.

17. Burgess A, van Diggele C, Roberts C, Mellis C. Tips for teaching procedural skills. BMC Med Educ. 2020;20:458.

18. Garcia-Rodriguez JA. Teaching medical procedures at your workplace. Can Fam Physician. 2016;62(4):351–54.

19. Sawyer T, White M, Zaveri P, Chang T, Ades A, French H et al. Learn, see, practice, prove, do, maintain: An evidence-based pedagogical framework for procedural skill training in medicine. Acad Med. 2015;90(8):1025–33.

20. Lacombe S, Forte M. Porcine procedure pads: How to build a teaching tool that's a cut above. Can Fam Physician. 2017;63(6):456–59.

21. Clarkson B, Telner D. Comprehensive dermatologic procedures pad: Innovation in hands-on resident procedural learning. Can Fam Physician. 2013;59(7):756–57.

22. Wetmore S. Defining competency-based evaluation objectives in family medicine: Procedure skills. Can Fam Physician. 2012;58(7):775–80.

23. Wass V, Archer J Assessing learners. In: Dornan T, Mann K, Scherpbier A, Spencer J (eds.), Medical education: Theories and practice. London: Churchill Livingstone; 2011.

24

Handling risk, uncertainty, and complexity

Helen Reid, Jenny Johnston, and Amanda Barnard

SUMMARY OF KEY LEARNING POINTS

- Clinical uncertainty and complexity are core aspects of family medicine (FM) and should be foundational learning within the undergraduate curriculum.

- Multiple complexities in FM, e.g. undifferentiated presentations, multimorbidity, and diverse social contexts of health, are intrinsically linked to clinical uncertainty.

- FM person-centred management, e.g. undifferentiated or evolving illness, complex decision-making, weighing risk, and outcomes, offers excellent learning opportunities.

- Managing uncertainty implies managing risk. This is a particularly uncomfortable and challenging aspect of practice for many learners in FM.

- Undergraduates must learn in the FM context to avoid overdiagnosis, investigation, and treatment as these in themselves risk potential iatrogenic harm to patients.

- Rural, remote, and resource-poor environments bring increasing clinical uncertainty, pushing family doctors to work at the margins of their scope of practice.

- The concept of "clinical courage" and other practical approaches can better equip learners to flourish alongside the uncertainty, complexity, and risk inherent in FM.

The challenge and opportunity of uncertainty

FM is privileged to sit close to individuals and communities across their unique contexts, offering solid healthcare foundations at a population level. The clinical generalism of FM offers intellectual stimulation, moral challenge, and values–based practice (Chapter 1). Yet its distinct paradigm of care may cause particular challenges for practitioners and learners more accustomed to secondary care, hospital-based medicine. Whereas hospital clinicians seek to increase clinical certainty, often through the use of tests, the role of family doctors is to accept uncertainty and manage risk safely as part of a complex clinical picture.

DOI: 10.1201/9781003325734-28

With many undergraduate curricula based largely in secondary care, students may have limited access to learning about these more ambiguous aspects of medicine. Those heading for work in FM may be underprepared for practice and its inherent uncertainty may even be perceived as a deterrent from pursuing careers within FM. For those destined for hospitalist careers, greater understanding of what happens on the "other side of the fence" can only be beneficial to communication across the primary–secondary care interface.

As academic family doctors, we argue that uncertainty, as part of the bedrock of FM, should be acknowledged within undergraduate curricula, and not left to postgraduate education.

Explicitly characterising the management of uncertainty as a fundamental skill amenable to development, rather than a threat, is crucial. This is key to unleashing the learning potential present in the FM context. Failure to address uncertainty with learners risks producing clinicians who are ill-equipped to face the realities of practice and are at increased risk of stress and burnout.[1]

> All medical students should graduate with an understanding of uncertainty and risk within an increasingly complex healthcare system. FM is an ideal context for learning these skills.

In this chapter, we define the term uncertainty, explore why it is of particular relevance in FM, and examine its relationship with complexity. We discuss the nature of risk in this context and suggest how to foster the "clinical courage" that will help medical students begin to learn how to manage risk safely. Throughout, we offer some practical suggestions for teaching about, and experientially alongside, these difficult concepts (Chapter 19).

Defining uncertainty

Uncertainty is a slippery concept. Arguably, humans are cognitively and emotionally hardwired to seek certainty. Indeed, the whole era of evidence-based practice, precision medicine, and artificial intelligence could be seen as a drive to increase diagnostic certainty in medicine.

After systematically reviewing articles addressing diagnostic uncertainty, Bhise et al. proposed defining it as a "subjective perception of an inability to provide an accurate explanation of the patient's health problem".[2] Yet, for family doctors, this cognitive approach to diagnosing uncertainty does not entirely make sense. Danczak and Lea propose a model supporting learners to understand and manage uncertainty based on actions. These are mapped against four key task areas—analysing, negotiating, networking, and team-working, as outlined in Figure 24.1.[3]

There are many other sources of uncertainty within FM, particularly around the more behavioural and affective challenges of working holistically with patients.

	Doctor/patient dyad	Team/family/ network	
D I A G N O S I S	*ANALYSE*	*NETWORK*	D I A G N O S I S
M A N A G E M E N T	*NEGOTIATE*	*TEAMWORK*	M A N A G E M E N T
	Doctor/patient dyad	Team/family/network	

FIGURE 24.1 Mapping uncertainty in medicine.

Paradoxically, uncertainty often increases as medicine advances with the development of more research, more available tests, and more drugs.

> Uncertainty goes beyond the ambiguity of diagnostic and management challenges to include reaction and negotiation with patients and colleagues.

Uncertainty is often perceived as particularly challenging for undergraduate learners in FM. Many students have been high achievers throughout their preceding education, always scoring well on assessments based on fact recall, knowing the "right" answers. An overreliance on incongruent assessments in many medical curricula (such as "single best answer" multichoice questions and narrow skills-based assessments set without suitable context) can further exacerbate the problem by failing to align with the intended learning (Chapter 27).

It is important to acknowledge that "naming" and openly discussing uncertainty will be more acceptable where there are cultural norms around patient–clinician shared decision-making. Amongst cultural groups where there is a hierarchical value expectation that "doctors should know", working and learning comfortably alongside uncertainty may be even more challenging for the trainee clinician (Chapters 12 and 22).

> Assessment cultures which rely on "single correct answers" or fail to align with intended learning may perpetuate an intolerance of uncertainty in learners.

Undifferentiated illness

In FM settings which offer primary healthcare, patients often present early in the development of their illness. They may be unclear about what they are suffering from, or if there is any connection between multiple symptoms. Their health beliefs and agendas may not necessarily align with the treating clinician's expectations. Through the give and take of complex relational care, clinicians undertake within the consultation a number of tasks of which forming a tentative diagnosis is often only one (Chapter 22). Scientific "knowledge", such as clinical guidelines, does suggest a comfortable degree of certainty, but the daily reality of FM presentations is that patients do not fit neatly into these boxes. Many FM practitioners deal with complex multimorbidity and will recognise how social determinants of health—inequalities, deprivation, and access to resources—are crucial factors in both health presentations and outcomes.

Complexity

Health and healthcare are inherently complex. Interactions between health determinants result in non-linear causal relationships with sometimes ambiguous outcomes. Context issues (such as the practicalities of accessing or delivering healthcare in some low- and middle-income countries) can render almost any health problem complex. Thus, in reality, complexity is intrinsic to all healthcare providers and learners in both specialist and generalist contexts. In many health systems, FM doctors care for the same patients at different stages of their life. Multimorbidity, a key contributor to complexity, is classically defined as the presence of two or more long-term medical conditions in an individual. It increases progressively with age. This matters due to the associations ageing brings with decreased quality of life, functional decline, and increased healthcare utilisation.[4]

> FM's proximity to undifferentiated illness and multimorbidity makes it an ideal setting for learning about complexity.

Complexity is inherent within the practice of modern medicine and all its paradigms. FM's proximity to undifferentiated illness and multimorbidity means we are

BOX 24.1 SUGGESTED PRACTICAL CURRICULAR STRATEGIES TO ADDRESS UNCERTAINTY AND COMPLEXITY WITH FM LEARNERS

- Formally integrate uncertainty into medical education curricula; discuss it, acknowledge it.
- Incorporate more "true to life" clinical learning such as case-based approaches.
- Build small-group learning sessions around single-disease management guidelines. Try applying findings to a patient who has this condition in addition to many others. Students could learn through presenting to each other.
- Support longitudinality in FM placements wherever possible—affording students opportunity to experience how time and continuity impact uncertainty.
- Promote forms of assessment which transcend "certain" or "right" answers (e.g. include workplace-based assessments [WPBAs]/entrustable professional activities [EPAs] rather than an overreliance on "single best answer" formats) (Chapter 27).

often balancing uncertainty when caring for an individual, whose management may not fit neatly, and with certainty, into disease-based clinical guidelines. This makes FM an ideal context to address clinical complexity with learners. Box 24.1 offers some suggested ways to embed uncertainty and complexity within the curriculum. Box 24.2 suggests some approaches for FM facilitators to support learning at clinical placement level.[5,6]

BOX 24.2 SUGGESTED PRACTICAL STRATEGIES TO ADDRESS UNCERTAINTY AND COMPLEXITY WITH FM LEARNERS AT INDIVIDUAL FM PLACEMENT FACILITATOR LEVEL

- Role model that it is "safe" and necessary to express uncertainty.
- Never be afraid to say, "I don't know", in response to a patient or student. These words invite curiosity, helping learners gain confidence in recognising where clinical uncertainty exists, and understand that communicating and sharing uncertainty is crucial.
- Promote curiosity over certainty by asking "How" and "Why" questions rather than "What" and "When".
- Identify patients with multimorbidity for FM students to see, focusing on their life and health experiences. How do they navigate local healthcare provision(s)? Do they have narratives showing how their care has been fragmented? Do they see multiple health professionals? What medications are they on, do they know what each one is for? What functional difficulties do they have?
- Encourage students to follow the course of individual patients' care, learning more about the natural history of disease and the potential benefit of time as a diagnostic tool in uncertain clinical presentations.

Risk

While some risks of potential harm to patients (e.g. medication interactions or surgeons mistakenly operating on the wrong side) can be mitigated by improvements at individual and system levels, patient safety can never be seen as absolute. Once a patient is approached holistically in a social context, the "greyness" in managing risk emerges. This is a defining feature of FM. Consider, for example, a harassed working mother who sometimes forgets her oral contraceptive pill and is at risk of pregnancy. Is an intrauterine device an option or is she happy to accept a small amount of risk? Thus, risk management becomes another core consultation task as the clinician and patient engage in shared decision-making and jointly negotiate an acceptable level of risk.

Another example of the social construction of risk management is managing an elderly person with anaemia who declines further investigation. In FM, especially, the risk exists of "missing" a significant diagnosis or opting for a management plan which results in a negative patient outcome. The FM practitioner's role is not, however, to investigate until certainty is achieved. The patient and doctor must reach a shared understanding of the degree of risk and agree on the level of uncertainty they can mutually tolerate.

There is a common misconception, particularly among medical students and junior postgraduate trainees, that risk must be mitigated by "more investigation" or "more referral" to specialist colleagues. Yet these strategies confer their own risks. Overdiagnosis and increased treatment burden are very real sources of iatrogenic harm, inadvertently caused through misguided approaches to dealing with risk. Medico-legal concerns around missing something important or choosing one management course over another are context dependent. Tolerance of risk is one of many factors at play when requesting diagnostic investigations. Not only will these vary with clinician experience and local accessibility, the health system structure (such as billing arrangements) is also highly relevant.

When uncertainty and complexity are high, risks will always be greater. Short supply of resources and time or difficulties with language and communication add additional complexity to healthcare encounters. In this sense, the coronavirus pandemic added multiple new layers of complexity to the work of family doctors worldwide.

> Students must learn to tolerate risk and avoid overinvestigation and unnecessary specialist referral as overdiagnosis and overtreatment are very real sources of iatrogenic harm.

Clinical courage

The term "clinical courage" has recently been used to describe how doctors respond to the challenges of working with uncertainty. This particularly applies when clinicians are pushed to the margins of their normal scope of practice. Early in the coronavirus pandemic, clinicians, and some students who experienced accelerated graduation into medical workforces, were forced to care for profoundly unwell patients with limited and varying resources and rapidly changing guidelines, often in areas outside their normal practice. They were frequently unable to delay care or defer to colleagues. We personally heard many stories from FM clinicians who, by necessity, moved to remote consulting and struggled to accommodate the extra complexity, uncertainty, and risk.

A definition of clinical courage is "that space where the needs of our patients and the extent of our training and experience intersect".[7] This concept is often applied to work in rural, remote, and low-resource settings. The challenges of the coronavirus pandemic and the demands it placed on clinicians across professions and all levels of experience made clinical courage a broader topical focus.[8]

> The coronavirus pandemic brought to the forefront the imperative to work with and despite uncertainty, challenging clinicians at the margins of their scope of practice.

Konkin et al. identified six features that characterise clinical courage in the work setting.[9] These are outlined in Box 24.3.

Internationally, the coronavirus pandemic challenged doctors to work at the very limits of their scope of practice. This created situations beyond their prior "tolerance of uncertainty" for diagnosis and management. We suggest the intuitive concept of clinical courage, and a more nuanced understanding of risk, and offer practical and accessible ways to help learners tolerate clinical uncertainty.

BOX 24.3 SIX FEATURES CHARACTERISING CLINICAL COURAGE IN THE WORKPLACE[9]

1. Standing up to serve anybody and everybody in the community.
2. Accepting uncertainty and persistently seeking to prepare.
3. Deliberately understanding and marshalling resources in the context.
4. Humbly seeking to know one's own limits.
5. Clearing the cognitive hurdle when something needs to be done for your patient.
6. Collegial support to stand up again.

Equipping FM learners to navigate risk and foster clinical courage

How might medical undergraduate education focus on providing the skills and understanding needed to equip students to working in environments at margins of their scope of practice? Ten Cate et al. suggest that creative problem-solving and adaptability, in the face of risk and uncertainty, require energy and initiative.[9]

The models of problem-based learning and medical apprenticeship can be structured to foster development of both reflection and self-regulated learning which support adaptive expertise ("the ability to apply knowledge adaptively and creatively").[10]

The term "safety netting" was introduced by Neighbour as a key strategy when managing risk.[11] This remains an important skill that all FM educators can seek to develop in learners (Chapter 22).

Safety netting comprises the following:

- Communication of uncertainty
- Advising what to look out for (including red flags)
- How to seek further help
- What time course to expect

Safety-netting is particularly important when risk and uncertainty are high, i.e. in the context of undifferentiated potentially serious presentations (febrile child) and patients at increased risk of complications (older patients, multimorbidity). The General Practice Supervisors Australia practical guide[12] offers well-explained practical aspects that FM educators might consider when supporting learners to handle risk. These include identifying patients' priorities and the judicious application of guidelines—"evidence-informed" practice.

> Exposing learners to challenging, unfamiliar cases to help them deliberately build problem-solving skills and deal with uncertainty and risk may serve to develop adaptive skills.

Conclusion

We have introduced the inevitability and interacting nature of uncertainty, complexity, and risk as they are experienced in FM. While not unique to learners in FM contexts, grappling with these issues is a daily reality in our clinical practice. We must face them head-on with our learners.

These concepts can seem abstract to students more used to tick-box accountability, but are a core element of professional development which should be introduced at undergraduate level. We offer suggestions for fostering undergraduate learners' skills to thrive alongside uncertainty, complexity, and risk. These include role modelling curiosity, careful attention to safety netting, and consideration of clinical courage.

References

1. Simpkin AL, Schwartzstein RM. Tolerating uncertainty: The next medical revolution? N Engl J Med. 2016;375(18):1713–5.

2. Bhise V, Rajan SS, Sittig DF, Morgan RO, Chaudhary P, Singh H. Defining and measuring diagnostic uncertainty in medicine: A systematic review. J Gen Intern Med. 2018;33(1):103–15.
3. Danczak A, Lea A. What do you do when you don't know what to do? GP associates in training (AiT) and their experiences of uncertainty. Educ Prim Care. 2014;25(6):321–6.
4. Wallace E, Salisbury C, Guthrie B, Lewis C, Fahey T, Smith SM. Managing patients with multimorbidity in primary care. BMJ. 2015;350:h176.
5. Gheihman G, Johnson M, Simpkin AL. Twelve tips for thriving in the face of clinical uncertainty. Med Teach. 2020;42(5):493–9.
6. Harding AHK, Rosenthal J. Learning general practice. A digital textbook for clinical students, postgraduate trainees, and primary care educators: Society for Academic Primary Care. Royal College of General Practitioners; 2021. Available from: www.ucl.ac.uk/epidemiology-health-care/sites/epidemiology_health_care/files/learning-general-practice.pdf
7. Wootton J. President's message. Clinical courage. Can J Rural Med. 2011;16(2):45–6.
8. Ten Cate O, Schultz K, Frank JR, Hennus MP, Ross S, Schumacher DJ et al. Questioning medical competence: Should the COVID-19 crisis affect the goals of medical education? Med Teach. 2021;43(7):817–23.
9. Konkin J, Grave L, Cockburn E, Couper I, Stewart RA, Campbell D et al. Exploration of rural physicians' lived experience of practising outside their usual scope of practice to provide access to essential medical care (clinical courage): An international phenomenological study. BMJ Open. 2020;10(8):e037705.
10. Lajoie SP, Gube M. Adaptive expertise in medical education: Accelerating learning trajectories by fostering self-regulated learning. Med Teach. 2018;40(8):809–12.
11. Neighbour R. The inner consultation: How to develop an effective and intuitive consulting style. 2nd ed. Boca Raton, FL: CRC Press; 2017.
12. Australia GPS. GP supervisor guide: Teaching skills in managing uncertainty; 2017. Available from: https://gpsupervisorsaustralia.org.au/wp-content/uploads/2017/04/Guide_Managing-Uncertainty_Digital.pdf

25

Well-being

Pramendra Prasad Gupta and Shelly B. Rodrigues

SUMMARY OF KEY LEARNING POINTS

- Family medicine (FM) is whole-person health. As holistic perspectives are fundamental to nurturing well-being, FM offers an excellent context for supporting medical students.
- Strong evidence of high levels of depression, anxiety, and burnout among students has led to medical schools becoming actively engaged in improving well-being and wellness.
- Well-being curricula, policies, and programmes are being integrated into education to support student awareness, faculty engagement, and administration requirements.
- Strategic curriculum design can support well-being by embedding opportunities to connect with each other—physical activity, ongoing learning, mindfulness, and giving.
- Many sources of leadership training literature support the work of faculty as they guide students, and other faculty members, towards well-being and wellness.
- FM faculty members can support medical student well-being and wellness by minding their own well-being and modelling techniques and activities to engage them in wellness.

Defining the problem

In recent years, and particularly since the recent COVID-19 pandemic, the need to address the well-being, wellness, and mental health of medical students has risen to the top of the education agenda. Research has been done in the United States, and globally, to learn more about the demands on medical students. The results have been troubling and have raised significant implications for future physicians. Wellness conferences and academic curricula have been developed to address

DOI: 10.1201/9781003325734-29

burnout and mental health. Professional organisations and specialty societies have prioritised these topic areas in their work.

> Family medicine is whole-person health and the whole-person concept extends to both physical and mental well-being and wellness.

Studies have shown a linkage between medical education and an erosion of mental health in medical students. A study in 2007, reported in the *Annals of Internal Medicine*, investigated a cohort of students across seven medical schools.[1] Of 4,287 participating students, 49.6% reported burnout and 11.2% of the respondents reported suicidal ideation. Research has also shown that medical students are three times more likely to commit suicide than the general population of the same age range. The prevalence of medical students screened for moderate to severe depression is high, while the willingness of these students to seek treatment is relatively low.

The COVID-19 pandemic has had a negative effect on all healthcare professionals. Medical students, in particular, have reported increased feelings of depression and anxiety and a decrease in available sources of support. In a study from Chaklader et al.,[2] 84.4% of all responding students reported that the pandemic had caused an increased sense of isolation from peers; 67.5% reported increased feelings of depression and 73% reported the same for anxiety.[2] These figures do not bode well for the well-being and wellness of the future medical workforce.

Burnout, the generic term used to describe the decreasing health well-being and wellness of professionals, has been studied as well. The Medscape National Physician Burnout and Depression Report for 2018, pre–COVID-19, surveyed 15,543 practising physicians from a variety of specialties; 23–48% reported burnout.[3] Medical student burnout rates are as high as those reported by practising physicians, with associated factors which include learner mistreatment, stress, and the high-stakes environment in which students learn.[3]

These findings, paired with negative outcomes for students as they struggle to care for themselves and their patients, clearly highlight a problem at all levels of medical education and training. Academic institutions and faculty members can address these factors.

> Well-being and wellness curricula, policies, and programmes are being integrated into medical education to support student awareness, faculty engagement, and administration requirements.

What is meant by well-being?

Well-being and wellness are frequently used interchangeably but should be differentiated. Well-being can be defined as a state of comfort, health, or happiness. Wellness is a state of being in good health. This includes social, physical, emotional, intellectual,

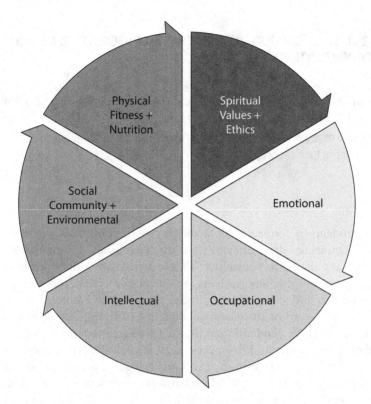

FIGURE 25.1 Balancing the aspects of personal health needed for an individual to be "well" and in a state of "well-being".

financial, and spiritual health (Figure 25.1). The aspects of personal health need to be balanced for an individual to be "well" and in a state of "well-being".

Addressing well-being in undergraduate education

While it may appear self-evident that good teaching alone will promote student mental well-being, a new range of work is now indirectly addressing well-being and wellness issues. A set of resources by Morgan and Houghton[4] identifies how to embed student and staff well-being as an important generic consideration for inclusive curriculum design. It suggests: "Considering which curriculum elements may cause stress or undue difficulties for particular students at the design stage enables course designers to structure modules and programmes in ways that will minimise the need for individual reasonable adjustments."[4]

Barnett[5] supports these concepts as well, identifying three connected fears that face students in a higher education context (Box 25.1).

What actions need to be taken to support the mental well-being of all students across a range of teaching contexts if these factors, plus the increase in burnout, depression, and anxiety, are to be addressed? The five ways to well-being by Steuer and Marks[6] provide one way of exploring the connection between learning and well-being. We now consider how each may be embedded in the learning and teaching context in FM.

BOX 25.1 THREE CONNECTED FEARS THAT FACE STUDENTS IN A HIGHER EDUCATION CONTEXT[5]

1. Fear of failure in a given task
2. Fear that one has fallen short of the role in which one has been cast and that one is not an authentic student
3. Fear of rejection as a person. This can affect well-being, paralysing a student, and restricting their capacity to learn

Connect

Enabling students to connect with faculty is crucial. This may be contingent on having a well-connected departmental team that establishes and maintains access points for students as a shared responsibility. This is particularly important in the context of large-group teaching, where students are out on placement and may be attached on their own to an FM clinic. Alternatively, they may feel isolated if they are in the minority (e.g. mature or international students) or living at home. As we move on from the COVID-19 pandemic environment where students became isolated from each other, from faculty and from patients, it is vital that we return to more blended learning and offer more face-to-face and small-group teaching[7] (Chapter 20).

It is important to identify any hidden barriers to connection that may exist. Students speak, for example, of their reluctance to talk with a faculty member about their difficulties and doubts as they may need to approach them for a job reference. Such reluctance may be increased on a professional programme where a student has a diagnosed mental, or other, health problem, and fears being judged "unfit" to practise.[8] Safe space must be established to ensure medical students feel able to access support.

> The COVID-19 pandemic has highlighted the importance of connecting with peers, patient, and faculty: Face-to-face interaction with peers, faculty, and patients contribute to student well-being.

Be active

Physical and mental well-being are closely linked. Providing opportunities for students to be active can encompass physical activity. Long periods of time spent immobile in claustrophobic teaching rooms can be stressful. Value is derived from thinking through how students can be encouraged to move around during or between teaching sessions, within the room or outside it. The needs of all students, including those with physical impairments, must be addressed.

Keep learning

A focus on "keeping learning" may seem self-evident within a higher education context where students have registered to read/study for a degree and graduate.

However, all students are likely to encounter factors that influence their confidence, motivation, and capacity to continue learning. Aspects of curriculum design, such as assessment and independent learning activities, can impact positively and negatively on learning processes. The importance of formative, constructive, personalised feedback is increasingly emphasised as a means for positively supporting students and encouraging action plans for ongoing learning (Chapter 28).

Take notice

Encouraging students to make and take notice of links between their own learning and what is going on in the world outside not only increases curriculum relevance, but also supports employability and internationalisation initiatives. It is important, too, for the promotion of well-being. We feel better when we are encouraged to take notice of the links between our learning and other aspects of our lives and relate it to the things we value. Taking notice can relate to looking inward as well as outward. Mindfulness approaches have been gaining ground within a higher education context.[9]

> Well-being can be built by enabling students to link their learning with all aspects of their lives—outwardly to global events around them and inwardly to their own personal values.

Contemplative pedagogy promoted by Barbezat and Bush[10] is a concept which encourages the integration of students' own lived experiences into learning. It enables them to develop a sense of connection with, and compassion for, others as well as deep thinking and problem-solving skills. It has been proposed as an antidote to the stresses of high-tech, multitasking environments.[11]

Give

Myriad opportunities exist for students to give to others while at university. Yet, all too often students perceive themselves as simply on the receiving end. Educators can address this by seeking ongoing feedback on their teaching, providing opportunities for students to shape both content and process, and encouraging students to help one another. "Service learning", and practice-based learning of other kinds, can provide opportunities for students to contribute to their wider community. It is important to provide feedback on, and where relevant thanks, for such contributions.

The Accreditation Council for Graduate Medical Education (ACGME) has been actively engaged in revising its requirements to address well-being and wellness. The 2017 requirements emphasise psychological, emotional, and physical well-being as critical to the development of "the competent, caring and resilient physician".[12] Walter Mills, former chair of the American Academy of Family Physicians' consultation on solutions for providing excellence in FM Residency Programmes, (https://www.afmrd.org/page/residency-program-solutions), recently highlighted to us that

BOX 25.2 FIVE PRACTICES THAT LEADERS MUST ENGAGE IN TO BE SUCCESSFUL[12]

Model the Way	Mirror well-being activities to students reflecting personal values
Inspire a Shared Vision	Develop goals that all involved own, care about, and work towards
Challenge the Process	Move outside the boundaries and engage in innovative activities
Enable Others to Act	Create a safe and trusting environment for people to collaborate, experiment, engage, and talk about fears and stresses
Encourage the Heart	Encourage students to work towards balance and seek wellness

well-being requires physicians to retain the "joy in medicine while managing their own real-life stresses". Retaining the joy of medicine must be modelled, learned, and nurtured.

FM faculty members can support medical student well-being by minding their own personal well-being and role modelling techniques and activities to engage in wellness.

Much of what we know about the burden of decreased well-being and wellness in medical students, residents-in-training, and physicians lies in the education and research literature. Leadership literature, in particular, holds key learnings for addressing the problem. In their leadership research, and subsequent work, Kouzes and Posner have identified five practices that leaders (mentors and faculty members can be included) must engage in to be successful[13] (see Box 25.2).

All five practices have important bearings for faculty members. Model the Way emphasises the importance of role modelling. It encourages leaders to mirror the way they ask others to behave and to reflect their own voice and values to them. The importance of role modelling practice clearly extends to faculty members as they deal with medical students' well-being and wellness. It is not enough to tell students to exercise, find balance, or do yoga. Faculty members should be powerful role models of wellness in their own lives. Kouzes and Posner[13] cite the last practice, "Encourage the Heart", as the one most lacking in leadership roles. We know that encouraging medical students to work towards balance and seek wellness is key to relieving the burden of burnout and nurturing a healthy medical and healthcare approach to learning.

Conclusion

There is compelling evidence, which medical education and faculty members need to acknowledge, that medical students are struggling with burnout and are reporting increased depression, anxiety, and suicidal ideation. This endangers the development of the future healthcare workforce. Resources and solutions are available to help transition to a medical education curriculum that supports students in both their clinical education and personal development. The evolution of medical education must emphasise psychological, emotional, and physical well-being as critical to the development of "the competent, caring and resilient physician". The words from the oath of Louis Lasagna,[14] read aloud to medical students during their white coat ceremonies, sum it up well:

> "I will remember that there is art to medicine as well as science, and that warmth, sympathy, and understanding may outweigh the surgeon's knife or the chemist's drug".[14]

References

1. Dyrbye LN, Thomas MR, Massie FS, Power DV, Eacker A, Harper W et al. Burnout and suicidal ideation among US medical students. Ann Intern Med. 2008;149:334–41.
2. Chakladar J et al. Medical students' perception of the COVID-10 pandemic effect on their education and well-being: A cross-sectional survey in the United States. BMC Med Educ. 2022;22:149. doi: 10.1186/s12909-022-03197-x
3. Medscape. Medscape national physician burnout and depressions report [Online]; 2018. Available from: https://www.medscape.come/slideshow/2018-lifestyle-burnout-depression-6009235#2
4. Morgan H, Houghton A. Inclusive curriculum design in higher education: Considerations for effective practice across and within subject areas [Internet]. New York: Higher Education Academy; 2011.
5. Barnett R. A will to learn: Being a student in an age of uncertainty. Maidenhead: Open University Press; 2007.
6. Steuer N, Marks N. University challenge: Towards a well-being approach to quality in higher education. London: New Economics Foundation; 2008.
7. Ardekani A, Hosseini SA, Tabari P, Rahimian Z, Feili A, Amini M et al. Student support systems for undergraduate medical students during the COVID-19 pandemic: A systematic narrative review of the literature. BMC Med Educ. 2021;21:352.
8. Stanley N, Ridley J, Manthorpe J, Harris J, Hurst A. Disclosing disability: Disabled students and practitioners in social work, nursing and teaching. London: Disability Rights Commission; 2007.
9. Bush M. Mindfulness in higher education. Contemp Buddhism. 2011;12(1):183–97.
10. Barbezat DP, Bush M. Contemplative practices in higher education: Powerful methods to transform teaching and learning. San Francisco: Jossey-Bass; 2014.
11. Levy DM, Wobbrock JO, Kaszniak AW, Ostergren M. Initial results from a study of the effects of meditation on multitasking performance: Extended abstracts of CHI; 2011. ACM Press.
12. Criteria for Excellence, 12th ed., Version 120.0, American Academy of Family Physicians and Residency Program Solutions. 2020:17–18.
13. KouzesJM, PosnerB. The leadership challenge. 5th ed. San Francisco: Jossey-Bass, John Wiley & Sons; 2012.
14. Sofia N, Alyssa B, Joe M, Vanessa K, Debashree S. Current directions in medical student wellbeing: A primer for students. Association of American Medical Colleges, Organization of Student Representatives. 2017.

26

Supervision, mentorship, and coaching

Oluseyi Akinola and David Keegan

SUMMARY OF KEY LEARNING POINTS

- Supervision, mentorship, and coaching should not be used interchangeably. There are subtle differences in purpose, intended outcomes, and the relationship between student and tutor.

- Effective supervisor and mentor relationships should build on trust established through clear expectations, guidelines, and accountability and a formative approach to learning.

- Family medicine (FM) offers a good context to supervise students across the curriculum given the breadth of generalist skills and the built-in holistic understanding of continuity of care.

- As FM physicians integrate into undergraduate education, they have increasingly important roles supervising students' activities and delivering formative and summative assessments.

- Mentoring in medical schools offers students personal support to nurture academic progress and well-being in a trusting confidential relationship with benefits for both mentor and mentee.

Definitions

Mentorship

Mentorship is the process whereby an experienced individual (the mentor) guides another individual (the mentee) in the development and reexamination of their own ideas, learning, and personal professional development.[1,2] It is a partnership built on confidence. Both partners need to work at sustaining the relationship.

DOI: 10.1201/9781003325734-30

Supervision

Supervision is the action or process of critical watching, stewardship, regulation of, and directing a course of activities or a course of action. A supervisor watches a learner do their work, provides feedback, and judges or grades the abilities of the learner.[2]

Coaching

Coaching is a supportive relationship in which a coach supports a coachee mainly by asking questions which help identify options for the coachee to pursue. A coachee may discuss a skill they have trouble accomplishing; the coach would ask questions to help the coachee develop their own plan for developing this skill.[3]

> While sometimes used interchangeably, it is important to understand the different roles of supervisors, mentors, and coaches.

The roles

Supervisors direct their learners' daily activities and set performance expectations. Their role is to get the job done, provide formative feedback, and make a judgement on how well a learner is performing.

Mentors are more trusted friends who guide career aspirations, provide a safe place for expressing concerns, and discuss uncomfortable and challenging scenarios. They act as soundboards for the mentee providing unbiased and confidential advice building on the mentee's strengths and weaknesses.

Coaches focus on the individual but are less directive and help the learner discover their own paths of learning and development.

Family physicians who are directly responsible for medical students' clinical learning, often on a 1:1 FM practice placement, can take on any of these roles, or even combine two or three effectively, within and/or outside direct clinical supervision. The FM generalist approach, from cradle to grave, enables them to be well vested in students' personal and professional growth and work–life balance to promote their well-being[3] (Chapter 25). Studies have emphasised the need for competency-based training (Chapter 10) and the importance of ongoing formative feedback (Chapter 28).

Hence the need for good mentors and supervisors who can take a holistic view of the student and their overall development as well-balanced future doctors. FM doctors, at the heart of primary care teams dealing with socially complex situations, are ideally suited to these roles. Integrating FM into the undergraduate curriculum offers students early exposure to a mentor or coach, who can understand their long-term interests and positively role model generalist practice exposing them to the real world and the life skills needed to thrive. This can help influence their career trajectory[4] (Chapter 15). Mentoring should be made available to all doctors, irrespective of the stage of their professional life.[5]

> FM physicians are well placed to supervise students on clinical placements and act as long-term personal tutors to role model skills needed to handle social complexity and real-life medicine.

Family physicians can inspire, communicate effectively, and demonstrate integrity, honesty, and consistency.[6] They can help medical students set important life goals and develop the skills to reach them by providing continuous feedback across the duration or defined time span of the relationship.[7] The aims of a mentoring relationship depend on the mentee's needs and can change over time as the mentee develops.[8] Successful mentorship is vital to career success for both mentees and mentors.[9,10] As students' experience of FM tends to be through supervision "within" longitudinal clinical placements or "without" through central campus mentoring in long-term personal tutor roles, we have chosen to focus on the roles of a supervisor and a mentor.

Global differences

As we set out to compare the processes of supervision and mentoring, we highlight the different perspectives we bring to this chapter and offer a personal experience, as outlined in Box 26.1.

BOX 26.1 A PERSONAL EXPERIENCE

Author OA has experience of studying at a low-middle income country (LMIC) medical school and residency postgraduate training in high-income Canada. The approach to mentoring and supervision across these settings was quite different. There are no formal structures in some LMICs for formal mentorship programmes. Emphasis is hierarchical with mentors being older individuals (Chapter 12). The roles and expectations of mentor and mentee tend to lack definition and are often hazy. The mentor's effectiveness depends on the type of direct life experiences shared with the mentee. In developed countries, where roles and expectations are clearly defined at the relationship's onset, the experience for OA became more relaxing with greater accountability and, most importantly, the development of trust. The fear as a medical student of public ridicule for wrong responses from the supervisor was dispelled the minute OA understood the ideal mentoring relationship was based on trust. Understanding that the feedback from her mentor was genuinely for her career growth, she started to flourish.

Unfortunately, many LMICs as yet lack reported examples of existing mentorship programmes.

> Effective supervisor and mentor relationships should build on trust established through clear expectations, guidelines, and accountability based on non-hierarchical value-based learning.

Supervision: Setting up

Supervisory roles are generally assigned to formal teaching relationships. It is critical for supervisors to understand their role and be aware of all performance expectations. The medical school should produce a guideline document with clear guidance on issues such as follows:

- Degrees of supervision to be provided to students at different stages.

- Practical examples of how to welcome learners into your clinical area.

- Processes in place to ensure student safety and well-being in learning environments.

- Clear learning outcomes and the methods used to assess students.

- How and when to assess the learner and give formative or summative feedback.

- The support provided by the medical school for supervisors.

- Reporting structures.

- What liability insurance coverage exists for the learner, if any.

Clear communication channels are essential. It is important before starting to understand the medical school processes in place for supervision and, should any concerns be raised, how to report if a student is struggling or to handle complaints (Chapter 30).

Supervising the learner at work: Directing and assessing activities

For novice medical students early in training, the supervisor becomes an important role model for observing FM doctors at work. They can be guided to understand generalist practice and holistic patient care. Observing students listening to patients' narratives before discussing issues related to their social history is a good place to start. As learners become more experienced, the principles of experiential learning (Chapter 19) can be used to design activities to give graded levels of increasing responsibility. The ultimate aim for high-performing medical students is an advanced apprenticeship level where they consult on their own while the supervisor remains at a distance but mindful of their direct clinical responsibility for patient care. This can be challenging for a supervisor.

The move to deliver and assess competency-based curricula (Chapters 10) will usually require supervisors to give regular formative feedback to progressively build learning. As highlighted, a safe learning environment where trust can be built enhances the supervisor's success in addressing students' strengths and weaknesses and any concerns they may have. Increasingly workplace-based assessment (WPBA) can require both formative and summative judgements (Chapter 27).

This can be very challenging in a 1:1 relationship with a student where collusion between supervisor and student can unconsciously develop. Tensions can exist between a student's high expectations of receiving good summative grades and a supervisor faced with the difficult task of delivering problematic formative advice and thus losing student confidence. Training supervisors to give feedback is essential (Chapter 28). It is important though to provide robust summative assessments on time to faculty and work formatively to identify struggling students (Chapter 30).

> Training supervisors to direct experiential learning activities and to formatively and summatively assess learning in 1:1 relationships is essential to ensure fair judgements and avoid collusion.

Mentorship

Mentorship relationships can follow different models.[1,2]

Apprenticeship model

The mentor has greater professional experience than the mentee. They can "sponsor" their mentee connecting them with opportunities to expand their professional network. For medical students, it may help secure electives.

Cloning model

The mentee is groomed to assume the role the mentor occupies. This can be used to develop leadership and service-focused roles.

Nurturing model

The mentor acts as a resource and facilitator guiding the mentee to education events and virtual collaboration forums, and/or review their work such as drafts of journal articles.

Peer mentoring model: The mentor and mentee are at the same level of training. They support each other to think through difficult scenarios and share opportunities and experiences. This model encourages and stimulates mutual growth as they relate well to each other at the same level of learning.

Globally, other mentoring models include the following:[14]

- *Formal mentoring:* Structured process supported by the institution or organisation.
- *Informal mentoring:* The relationship is developed between parties involved.

Instrumental mentoring: Here, the instrumental mentor serves as a coach and an advisor, helping the protégé negotiate the environment and mostly based on the direct life experiences of the mentor.

Traditionally, the mentoring relationship is one-on-one chosen by the mentor and mentee or, in medical schools where student cohorts can be large, allocated. They can be formal, with a rigid structure and process, or informal, with irregularly timed meetings and less structure. Increasingly, via the use of technology solutions (emails, Zoom, Microsoft Teams), distance mentoring has emerged and has been strengthened by the COVID-19 pandemic. An alternative is group mentoring where a single mentor directs the activities of a group of mentees with similar interests and objectives.

Most medical students agree that a mentor is important for psychosocial support and future career planning, with the need greatest as they approach graduation.[11] The mentor's main role is to create a safe and open environment where the mentee feels heard, free of bias and judgement, and can openly discuss personal and professional issues. A mentee can seek out a mentor.[12] Mentees, as highlighted above, are encouraged to raise difficult issues, and discard hierarchical discomforts to focus on proactive learning and receiving objective feedback (not defensive) with a positive attitude. Awareness of sociocultural differences and potential conflicts of interest is important. Mentors should enable the mentee to learn and explore options for themselves.

> Personal mentors are increasingly allocated in medical schools to support students to share difficult issues in a safe confidential environment. FM doctors are well placed to take this role.

Outcomes are generally confidential and not reported to faculty. Challenges can arise for the mentor when a student has a serious issue such as mental health problems or family crises. They can be reluctant to report this (Chapter 25) and the skills of the mentor come into play in negotiating a mutually acceptable resolution. The medical schools may require periodic reviews to monitor progress of initial objectives set by the mentorship team.

The mentor therefore needs certain attributes to be effective (see Box 26.2) and specific training from the medical school to be aware of the curriculum, faculty expectations, student assessment, and programme evaluation processes.

The benefits of mentorship

The role of mentorship and supervision for learners in FM is invaluable. It enables mentees to gain practical knowledge and insight from experienced generalist physicians and offers mentors the opportunity to update their professional knowledge and refine their skills. The full benefits are summarised in Table 26.1.[1,13]

FM, as a generalist specialty, cuts across the breadth of the lifespan, from cradle to grave, and offers holistic continuity of care. This mirrors the role of the mentor in enhancing, supporting, and facilitating the mentee to take responsibility for their own growth and self-development to enhance their knowledge base and skill sets.

BOX 26.2 ATTRIBUTES REQUIRED OF AN EFFECTIVE MENTOR

An effective mentor must be able to do the following:

- Listen actively
- Set well-defined achievable goals
- Question effectively
- Demonstrate empathy
- Check understanding
- Give constructive feedback
- Build trusting non-hierarchical relationships
- Respect confidentiality
- Motivate continuous improvement
- Manage time well

The mentor is helping the mentee unlock their potential to maximise their own performance by sharing their own knowledge, skill, and experience.

The breadth of FM generalist skills and holistic approach to relationships bring important attributes to student mentoring provided the medical school's expectations of mentors are clear.

TABLE 26.1 The benefits of mentorship for the mentor and mentee

Mentee	Mentor
Career coaching and support	Personal gratification and fulfilment
Professional stimulation to achieve career goals	Learning opportunity, an opportunity to acquire CPD requirements /credits
Research guidance and collaboration	Improve skills: active listening, interpersonal communication, and actively building trust
Guidance on promotion and tenure	Strengthens knowledge
Networking opportunities	Builds confidence
Decreased burnout	Improves job satisfaction
Access to resources for knowledge and skills	Opportunity for self-reflection
Encourages accountability	Gains new perspectives
Useful and constructive feedback	Establishes leadership skills
Access to a free resource	Enhances one's resume and network

There are clear benefits for institutions through increased faculty retention, commitment to the development of the next generation of leaders in academic medicine, and the potential for increased research output.[5,11,14]

Conclusion

FM is a lifelong art of continuous and comprehensive healthcare delivery to patients from cradle to grave. It is complex, challenging, and rewarding requiring each of us to be a mentee or mentor every day. A good mentor or supervisor in undergraduate medical education is pivotal to ensuring all graduates, whatever career they ultimately aspire to, are well-trained and well-rounded with coping skills to navigate the challenges of life and career, creating a good work–life balance and overall well-being.

An effective mentor has an altruistic personality,[9] demonstrates integrity and honesty, maintains confidentiality, and is respectful of the mentee at all times. It is our hope that FM supervisors and mentors globally can embrace this culture shift and cultivate a trust-based relationship of active, empathic listening to medical students. If in a supervisory role, encouraging self-reflection and delivering regular constructive feedback is of paramount importance to identify learners who are underperforming and ensure earlier remediation can be arranged.

References

1. Ratnapalan S. Mentoring in medicine. Can Fam Physician. 2010;56(2):198.
2. Hernandez-Lee J, Pieroway A. Mentorship for early career family physicians. Can Fam Physician. 2018;64:861.
3. En Toh RQ, Koh KK, Lua JK, Wong RSM, Quah ELY, Panda A et al. The role of mentoring, supervision, coaching, teaching and instruction on professional identity formation: A systematic scoping review. BMC Medical Educ. 2022;10(22):1. doi: 1186/s12909-022-03589-z
4. Strauss SE, Chatur F, Taylor M. Issues in the mentor–mentee relationship in academic medicine: A qualitative study. Acad Med. 2009;84(1):135–39.
5. Macleod S. The challenge of providing mentorship in primary care. Postdrad Med J. 2002;83(979):317–9.
6. Jordan J, Watcha D, Cassella MSC, Trivedi S. Impact of a mentorship program on medical student burnout. 2019;3(3):218–5. doi: 10.1002/aet2.10354
7. Russell JEA. The changing nature of mentoring in organizations: An introduction to the special issue on mentoring in organizations. J Vocational Behavior. 1997;51(1):1–14. doi: 10.1006/jvbe.1997.1602
8. Taherian K, Skekarchian M. Mentoring for doctors. Do its benefits outweigh disadvantages? Med Teach. 2008;30(4):e95–e9.
9. Straus SE, Johnson MO, Marquez C, Feldman MD. Characteristics of successful and failed mentoring relationships: A qualitative study across two academic health centers. Acad Med. 2013;88(1):82–9.
10. Fallatah HI, Soo Park Y, Farsi J, Tekian A. Mentoring clinical-year medical students: Factors contributing to effective mentoring. J Med Educ Curric Dev. 2018;5. doi: 10.1177/2382120518757717

11. Association of American Medical Colleges. Five tips for finding and working with a mentor. https://students-residents.aamc.org/choosing-medical-career/5-tips-finding-and-working-mentor. Students & residents. Available from: https://students-residents.aamc.org/choosing-medical-career/5-tips-finding-and-working-mentor (Accessed 1 February 23).

12. Canadian Medical Association. Mentorship in health care. Available from: https://www.cma.ca/physician-wellness-hub/topics/mentorship (Last accessed 1 February 23).

13. University of Toronto. Diversity mentorship programme for under-represented or minoritized medical students and first-year residents. Available from: https://temertymedicine.utoronto.ca/diversity-mentorship-program (Accessed 1 February 23).

14. Onyeonoru I, Okoli-Ikedi O, Nweke J, Ahmadu F. Mentoring in a Nigerian university: An analysis of mentor–protégée relationship and benefits. Niger J Sociol Anthropol. 2016;14. doi: 10.36108/NJSA/6102/14(0230)

Assessment

Assess it, and it becomes important. Assess it explicitly ... with transparent criteria, and perhaps they will see why.

Peter James

Assessing clinical competency

Mohamed Hany Shehata and Marwa Mostafa Ahmed

SUMMARY OF KEY LEARNING POINTS

- Clinical competency is the ability of students to apply complex combinations of knowledge, skills, and attitudes for safe and effective unsupervised clinical practice.
- Undergraduate training in family medicine (FM) provides an excellent opportunity to learn multiple competencies in a safe supervised environment.
- Formative assessment of competencies in FM rotations necessitates the use of multiple workplace based assessment (WPBA) tools with constructive feedback.
- When placed in FM contexts, students should be given every opportunity to manage patients under direct supervision followed by formative feedback from experienced trainers.
- Modern competency-based assessment is achievement based rather than time based. Learners' capacity for self-assessment tends to be unreliable.
- Objective Structured Clinical Examinations (OSCEs) provide a reliable method of summative assessment for undergraduate training in FM.

Competency-based medical education

We define competency as "a physician's ability to apply complex combinations of knowledge, skills, and attitudes for safe and effective unsupervised clinical practice". Competency-Based Medical Education (CBME) offers an outcome-based training which ensures that on graduation students have the required competencies to deliver safe and better medical care (Chapter 10). Traditionally, medical school assessments have been *summative* through end of course examinations designed to measure whether a student is safe to progress and under threat of failure. CBME has moved curricula towards *formative* assessment, i.e., measuring and giving constructive, non-threatening feedback to improve students' performance during the course (Chapter 28).[1]

DOI: 10.1201/9781003325734-32

A competence-based undergraduate curriculum starts by defining learning outcomes which are then adopted to design, implement, and monitor the educational programme. When assessing students, CBME has the advantage of highlighting the need to constructively align the clinical and educational outcomes with appropriate assessment methodology. This provides greater flexibility and accountability across the curriculum. To improve healthcare quality and ensure patient safety, CBME should be implemented throughout undergraduate and postgraduate medical education and continuing professional development. This supports the continuous development of a doctor's ability to integrate knowledge, skills, and attitudes within their competencies as they move along the novice to expert pathway.[2]

> In a CBME curriculum, formative and summative assessment methodologies must be carefully selected to constructively align with the learning outcomes.

Alignment of assessment with family medicine training

In undergraduate education, FM provides an excellent opportunity for students to receive comprehensive integrated training on multiple competencies under supervision. This should now be integrated into all modern undergraduate programmes. Early exposure of medical students to patients typically takes place in primary healthcare centres (PHCs) in various community settings[3,4] (Chapter 15). Sending students to learn in PHCs usually aims to not only enrich their clinical skills but also to foster other essential competencies, as outlined in Box 27.1.

Globally, medical schools are introducing FM clerkship(s) of varying length, often in later years nearer graduation. The focus shifts to clinical competencies best learnt in the generalist context of primary care, e.g. undifferentiated diagnosis, multi-comorbidity, and complex management. FM clerkships provide students with comprehensive clinical training offering opportunities, not necessarily available in secondary care, to teach and formatively assess these generalist competencies.

BOX 27.1 EXAMPLES OF COMPETENCIES WHICH CAN BE LEARNT IN FM

- Community orientation and awareness of priority health-related problems
- Communication with patients and colleagues
- Collaboration with colleagues and healthcare providers (interprofessional)
- Preventive aspects of healthcare and evidence-based health maintenance
- Awareness of the healthcare system and its delivery of quality healthcare
- Ethics and professionalism
- Quality improvement and patient safety
- Community-oriented research

Applying CBME in FM carries opportunities and threats. The competency-based framework, supported by 1:1 supervision from FM doctors in the safe environment of small professional teams, provides student-centred clinical training and constructive formative feedback (Chapter 28). Yet, often in early years, assessments are summative and campus based using methods which fail to align with community-intended learning outcomes (Box 27.1). An important threat in later years is losing the comprehensive holistic FM approach. This is driven by fragmentation of over-complex specialist care outcomes into measurable competencies.[5] Inevitably, assessment drives learning. Unless visibly assessed, students can marginalise community learning.

> FM provides a safe learning environment with the tutor supervision needed to assess students formatively. Generalist outcomes risk marginalisation unless explicitly assessed.

Comprehensive competency-based assessment

Careful selection of summative, e.g., applied knowledge tests, OSCEs, and formative methods, e.g. WPBAs and portfolios, is essential to assess FM learning outcomes effectively and explicitly (Chapter 29). All "stakeholders", including faculty interprofessional team members, real and simulated patients, and other healthcare providers should have input. It is important to explicitly engage and empower students. Understanding these factors, and how they interact, is important for designing, implementing, and constantly improving a comprehensive competency-based assessment system.[6]

Student activities in community-based training (CBT) require careful selection of assessment tools to explicitly align with the intended learning. Shewade et al. have developed a self-assessment tool for CBT.[7] This covers several domains: public health (epidemiology and research methods), biostatistics, healthcare service delivery, FM, community development, and generic or cultural competencies.[7]

Assessing clinical competency

Assessing clinical competencies in FM to ensure reliable measurement across different clinical situations, and during real performance, is challenging. CBME focuses on the learner's ability which is context-specific, i.e. it varies across different situations. Because of the integrated nature of competency, discrepancies arise between a student's ability to perform in different authentic clinical contexts. This is challenging given the breadth and depth of FM. Clinical encounters are often less well defined in comparison to secondary care. Students need to apply their knowledge to undifferentiated presentations using clinical reasoning and decision-making skills in a professional manner (Chapter 21).

For example, a student may be a competent communicator and know how to diagnose and manage a child with eczema but may not transfer these skills and communicate effectively when faced with an elderly patient with diabetes. Managing patients with several chronic illnesses can challenge students who can no longer rely solely on single-disease-based knowledge accrued on hospital specialty rotations. Utilising their knowledge and communication skills to provide a patient-centred plan that enhances an asthmatic adolescent's self-care or addresses an obese diabetic patient's non-adherence to a management plan is crucial learning in the FM holistic context. Such rich encounters provide excellent formative opportunities for "assessment for learning". Clinical tutors can provide 1:1 supervision of students managing these cases and utilise WPBA assessment tools to feedback constructively encouraging students to identify their gaps and how to improve and close these. This approach builds authentic student-centred clinical competency.

> Competencies are context-specific not generic. In FM, this can challenge students faced with the breadth and depth of undifferentiated patient presentations.

Integrating summative and formative assessment is crucial to the development of competencies through deliberate practice. Using various assessment tools helps students identify their strengths and weaknesses and enhances the validity and reliability of the assessment. In a study conducted in Saudi Arabia,[8] comprehensive assessment of medical students during FM training was used to measure different skills and levels of competency according to Miller's pyramid (Chapter 29).[9] Integration of applied knowledge tests (including single best answer [SBA] and extended matching multichoice questions [MCQs] and OSCEs were used to assess the "Knows", "Knows how", and "Shows how") levels of Miller's pyramid.[9] Comprehensive assessment throughout the course measured the "Does" level. Results showed significant positive correlations, which reflected the actual student performance, between all assessment methods.[8]

In multiple studies, WPBA tools have proved to have excellent utility when used in undergraduate clinical assessment. In one study, the mini-clinical evaluation (mini-CEX) emerged as a promising formative and summative assessment method which was reasonably valid, reliable, acceptable, and feasible. In this study, the mini-CEX had a satisfactory educational impact resulting from structured observation and feedback.[10] Farajpour et al. concluded that direct observation of procedural skills (DOPs) provides feasible and valid assessment which ensures adequate medical student learning assessing their readiness for accepting professional responsibilities.[11] There is a lack of published research work on the use of case-based discussions (CbDs) in undergraduate medical education. However, this method permits constructive decision-making with a tutor in the undifferentiated FM context and has potential.

> Integration of formative and summative assessment methods in FM markedly improves the validity and reliability of assessing medical students on generalist competencies.

Mentoring and constructive feedback

Mentoring and providing personalised, timely, constructive feedback are powerful tools and should be integrated into any system assessing competency (Chapters 26 and 28). Simulation can provide immediate assessment and feedback in a less threatening environment. It protects the patients from any harm until students feel confident to interact directly with them. Simulation and role-play (especially for common FM procedural and communication competencies), using mastery-based standards, should be implemented alongside a combination of WPBAs.[6]

FM training provides a perfect medium for role modelling by experienced tutors who are trained to mentor and nurture student development. Specific faculty development is needed to ensure the continuous capacity-building of trainers.

> Simulating patients through role play is a powerful learning and assessment tool if supervised by FM tutors trained to give constructive feedback.

Formative assessment on community attachments can focus on FM-orientated skills (Box 27.1) and the holistic patient-centred management of comorbidity and undifferentiated presentations. Using different WPBA tools, such as direct observation, multi-source feedback, patient experience surveys, and CbD, strengthens assessment across the range of FM competencies. For summative assessment, often medical school campus based, it is important family physicians exam in OSCEs and write items to support the integration and contextualisation of FM into the questions to make it explicit to students that learning in FM matters.

> Investing in faculty development is important for improving teaching, feedback, assessment, and coaching skills and for progressing their roles in the medical school.

Active engagement by the student

Assessing clinical competencies requires active involvement and empowerment of students in the assessment process. Students should be encouraged to adopt the concept of "self-directed assessment seeking".[6] Formal summative assessments, e.g. OSCEs, provide opportunities for students to accurately rate their competence, but detailed constructive feedback on how to improve is not often given. Unfortunately, self-assessment of competence risks inaccuracy. A study from India assessed students' self-predictions of their competence pre and post a FM OSCE and compared their ratings with the OSCE marks. Before the OSCE, students were unable to predict their level of competence while after the exam their self-assessment levels decreased. The self-ratings correlated poorly with their actual performance.[12] This is consistent with other published findings and represents an obstacle to self-paced learning in competency-based FM education.[13] Multiple tools, such as portfolios and reflective diaries can encourage students to reflect on their own performance.[14]

> Self-assessment can be unreliable—good students underestimating and poor students overestimating their ability. Self-reflection using portfolios and diaries should be encouraged.

Milestones and entrustable professional activities

Milestones are behavioural descriptions of the ability expected from students as they progress through the curriculum. Detailed milestones act as benchmarks against which students' performance is assessed. They guide selection of suitable assessment tools and enable students to track progress towards appropriate levels of competence.[14,15]

Entrustable professional activities (EPAs) are emerging as a method for judging competency. The core clinical activities expected of a medical student are defined and scaled to the level of experience.[16] EPAs integrate the required clinical competencies into more comprehensive, observable, and measurable activities used to assess the student's ability. A certain defined task can be fully entrusted to a student if they have successfully performed at the competence level required to perform the activity in clinical practice. Construction of detailed descriptions of EPAs to define exactly what is expected from the student entrusted with a task at each milestone is important for their successful implementation in a CBME programme.[16]

Training assessors to be better assessors and accurate observers of clinical competencies is mandatory, especially during authentic patient care in primary healthcare centres. Different interactions are present that cannot be simulated and assessed with simulated patients.[6]

Conclusion

Assessing core clinical competencies in FM and ensuring students can demonstrate these in practice is challenging yet crucial. Figure 27.1 summarises the essential components underpinning successful assessment of competency in clinical practice.

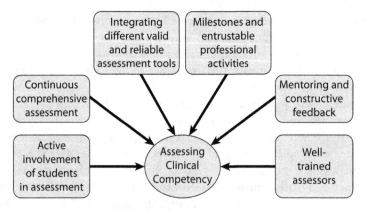

FIGURE 27.1 Programmatic assessment of clinical competency.

A robust system integrates various assessment methods and actively engages students in the process. Providing personalised constructive feedback and developing detailed milestones are powerful tools that should be integrated across the programme. Investing in faculty development is mandatory to train tutors to be more precise observers and better judges of student performance.

References

1. Lochnan H, Kitto S, Danilovich N et al. Conceptualization of competency-based medical education terminology in family medicine postgraduate medical education and continuing professional development: A scoping review. Acad Med. 2020;95(7):1106–19. doi: 10.1097/ACM.0000000000003178

2. Kruse J. Social accountability across the continuum of medical education: A call for common missions for professional, accreditation, certification, and licensure organizations. Fam Med. 2013;45:208–11.

3. Institute of Medicine (US) Committee on the Future of Primary Care; Donaldson MS, Yordy KD, Lohr KN et al. (eds.). Primary care: America's health in a new era. Washington, DC: National Academies Press; 1996. Education and Training for Primary Care. p. 7. https://www.ncbi.nlm.nih.gov/books/NBK232645/

4. Magzoub ME, Schmidt HG. A taxonomy of community-based medical education. Acad Med. 2000;75(7):699–707. doi: 10.1097/00001888-200007000-00011

5. Schneider B, Biagioli FE, Palmer R, O'Neill P, Robinson SC, Cantone RE. Design and implementation of a competency-based family medicine clerkship curriculum. Fam Med. 2019;51(3):234–40. doi: 10.22454/FamMed.2019.539833

6. Holombe ES, Sherbino J, Long DM, Swing SR, Frank JR. The role of assessment in competency-based medical education. Med Teach. 2010;32(8):676–82. doi: 10.3109/0142159X.2010.500704

7. Shewade HD, Jeyashree K, Kalaiselvi S, Palanivel C, Panigrahi KC. Competency-based tool for evaluation of community-based training in undergraduate medical education in India: A Delphi approach. Adv Med Educ Pract. 2017;8:277–86. doi: 10.2147/AMEP.S123840

8. AlShamlan NA, Al Shammari MA, Darwish MA, Sebiany AM, Sabra AA, Alalmaie SM. Evaluation of multifaceted assessment of the fifth-year medical students in family medicine clerkship, Saudi Arabia experience. J Multidiscip Healthc. 2020;13:321–28. doi: 10.2147/JMDH.S241586

9. Miller GE. The assessment of clinical skills/competence/performance. Acad Med. 1990;65(9):S63–S7. doi: 10.1097/00001888-199009000-00045.

10. Hejri SM, Jalili M, Masoomi R, Shirazi M, Nedjat S, Norcini J. The utility of mini-clinical evaluation exercise in undergraduate and postgraduate medical education: A BEME review: BEME Guide no. 59. Med Teach. 2020;42(2):125–42. doi: 10.1080/0142159X.2019.1652732

11. Farajpour A, Amini M, Pishbin E, Mostafavian Z, Akbari Farmad S. Using modified direct observation of procedural skills (DOPS) to assess undergraduate medical students. J Adv Med Educ Prof. 2018;6(3):130–36.

12. Graves L, Lalla L, Young M. Evaluation of perceived and actual competency in a family medicine objective structured clinical examination. Can Fam Physician. 2017;63(4):e238–e43.

13. Yates N, Gough S, Brazil V. Self-assessment: With all its limitations, why are we still measuring and teaching it? Lessons from a scoping review. Med Teach. 2022. doi: 10.1080/0142159X.2022.2093704

14. Holmboe ES. The transformational path ahead: Competency-based medical education in family medicine. Fam Med. 2021;53:583–89.
15. Dhaliwal U, Gupta P, Singh T. Entrustable professional activities: Teaching and assessing clinical competence. Indian Pediatr. 2015;52(7):591–97. doi: 10.1007/s13312-015-0681-3
16. Ten Cate O, Taylor DR. The recommended description of an entrustable professional activity: AMEE Guide no.140. Med Teach. 2021;43(10):1106–14. doi: 10.1080/0142159X. 2020.1838465

28

The principles of feedback

Chris Harrison and Hashmet Parveen

SUMMARY OF KEY LEARNING POINTS

- Feedback can be a very powerful tool but often fails to reach its potential.
- Overreliance on rigid "feedback formulae" is often unhelpful.
- Guidelines on feedback need to be interpreted with flexibility and tailored to the individual learner.
- A balance needs to be struck between supporting the student while still tackling challenging issues.
- Feedback needs to be viewed as a meaningful conversation between tutor and student, not as a formulaic one-way delivery mechanism.

Defining feedback

Feedback is one of the most important aspects of education, yet it is frequently misunderstood. It is typically defined as follows:

> Specific information about the comparison between a trainee's [student's] observed performance and a standard, given with the intent to improve the trainee's performance.[1]

It is worthwhile taking some time to reflect on each part of the definition. Feedback can be an extremely powerful and positive phenomenon, having a significant impact on a student's learning. However, feedback often fails to reach its potential and does not always lead to improvements in performance. In this chapter, we will explore some of the reasons for this, and develop some practical tips to help feedback work better for you and your learners.

DOI: 10.1201/9781003325734-33

The importance of observation

At the most fundamental level, it is obviously vital that practitioners observe their learners working in the clinical workplace. It might seem unnecessary to say this, but in busy clinical environments, pressure of work has often resulted in learners only being directly observed on a very infrequent basis. However, learners will not usually regard your feedback as credible if you are relying on indirect information about them.[2] We cannot emphasise enough the importance of setting aside time on a regular basis to observe the authentic performance of your students first-hand. Students appreciate being actively involved in a consultation, rather than just passively observing a tutor at work.

> It's vital to make time to regularly observe your student working authentically in the clinical workplace.

As implied in the definition above, the observation needs to be purposeful, comparing the learner's performance with the expected standard or milestone (Chapter 27). It is imperative that you have a clear understanding of the standards set for a student to achieve at their level of training. To help structure your observations, many medical schools will give you a checklist or guide. At one extreme, these are dominated by multiple grading opportunities, with little space for narrative feedback, whereas at the other extreme, they are focused simply on whether the student can achieve the desired outcome. As outlined in Chapter 27, some structure using workplace-based assessment tools (WPBA) can be helpful to guide the observation, e.g. into different parts of the consultation, but an over-rigid structure is usually counterproductive. We will discuss the problem with grades later in this chapter.

> Feedback guidelines need to be interpreted with flexibility.

Is there a magic formula to help you give feedback?

Over the years, various "feedback formulae" have been devised, each with their various supporters. Well-known models include the "Feedback Sandwich",[3] Pendleton's Model,[4] Agenda-Led Outcome-Based Analysis (ALOBA),[4] and R2C2.[5] More details are provided in Box 28.1.

There are some common, recurring features, such as the need to balance positive, reinforcing comments with more critical or corrective ones. These formulae can be helpful to guide practitioners in the early stages of learning about feedback but need to be applied with caution as their use can be problematic.

BOX 28.1 EXAMPLES OF FEEDBACK FORMULAE

The Feedback Sandwich:[3]
- Praise a specific part of the consultation that was done well
- Criticise a specific part of the consultation that could be improved
- Praise another specific part of the consultation that was done well

Pendleton's Model:[4]
- Briefly clarify matters of fact.
- The learner describes what was done well, and how.
- The tutor says what was done well, and how.
- The learner describes what could have been done differently, and how.
- The tutor says what could have been done differently, and how.

Agenda-Led, Outcome-Based Analysis (ALOBA)[4]
- Start with the learner's agenda.
- Look at the outcomes the learner and patient are trying to achieve.
- Encourage self-assessment and self-problem-solving first.
- Use descriptive feedback to encourage a non-judgemental approach.
- Provide balanced feedback.
- Make offers and suggestions, generate alternatives.
- Rehearse suggestions.
- Be well-intentioned, valuing, and supportive.
- Structure and summarise learning so that a constructive endpoint is reached.

R2C2 Model:[5]
- Relationship building
- Exploring Reactions to the feedback
- Exploring understanding of feedback Content
- Coaching for performance change

Problems with feedback

Avoid being over formulaic

One of the main problems with following a feedback formula is that it can lead to a rigid and stilted discussion. The tutor is often strongly in control while the student is much more passive. If the tutor is following a formula strictly, they cannot deal with a student's concerns at the time they are raised as these need to be addressed at a different step in the formula. When students are used to a particular formula, they can find it very repetitive. For example, they may often ignore the positive opening parts of the feedback sandwich while waiting for delivery of the "meat".

Multiple factors play a role in the interpretation and uptake of feedback.

The natural desire to be supportive to learners can lead to doctors avoiding difficult areas in the feedback discussion. Instead, they concentrate on praising the student. This can amount to a form of collusion with the student, in much the same way that family doctors can collude with patients to avoid challenging issues in order to remain well-liked. Although this is a very understandable temptation, we need to remember that the feedback definition requires us to try to improve the student's performance. There is often a balance to be struck between remaining popular with the students and ensuring performance improves, although the strength of each factor may vary according to different cultural norms. A paper by Boehler et al. demonstrated that giving compliments, without highlighting areas to work on, can lead to high levels of student satisfaction but does not improve clinical skills performance.[6] Of course, we are *not* advocating that doctors should completely abandon their encouraging, supportive approach for a negative, destructive attitude which is likely to be detrimental for the tutor–student relationship.

Feedback needs to be timely, and trainers need to be credible role models.

Avoid grades, be specific, and use narrative

Intrinsic to the feedback definition is the requirement to provide *specific* information. Feedback is often too general to instigate change in a student's behaviour or tends to focus on the student's personality rather than their observed behaviours or skills. Students can find this very frustrating.[7] In a similar way, grades can be problematical. On the one hand, grades provide some clarity and reassurance to learners about the expected level of performance. On the other hand, grades without narrative feedback fail to provide students with sufficient information to stimulate improvement. Students are often so used to grades that, at first, they find the lack of them disconcerting. However, as they become used to more narrative feedback, they develop a more nuanced view of their own strengths and weaknesses. The lack of reassurance from "good enough" grades incentivises them to aspire towards excellence.[7]

Avoid grading performance. Narrative on how to improve is important to stimulate all students to aim for excellence.

Avoid information overload

Although the need to be specific is very important, this does not mean that you should feel that you have to tell the learner everything. There is a danger of feedback overload. It is important to choose the most important and relevant issues that need to be fed back on each particular occasion. Students frequently prefer verbal to written feedback, although tutors find that the need to prepare written feedback can improve the quality of their verbal feedback.[8]

Respect the individuality of the learner

Perhaps the most fundamental problem when delivering feedback is an assumption that "one size fits all". Learners naturally vary enormously in their strengths and weaknesses and in the desire for more supportive versus more challenging feedback. Rather than focusing on a formula for *delivering* feedback to all learners, it is therefore vital to consider how the feedback will be *received*. Instead of a feedback monologue, it's important to have a meaningful conversation with your learners. There is strong evidence that this leads to much better outcomes.[9]

Do not deliver feedback in the same way to all learners: one size does not fit all.

Both the learner and the tutor need to be invested in the conversation, prepared to listen and consider other perspectives. In many ways, it can be considered analogous to a patient–centred consultation in family practice, where there is a need for attentive listening, empathy, and negotiation.[10] Take care with the language you use to ensure mutual respect and understanding. Feedback is inevitably subjective, but this is nothing to fear. To take another analogy, we can all hold different but valuable perspectives on a piece of artwork, but it is usually possible to find some common ground.

Feedback needs to be delivered in a timely manner, ideally immediately after a period of observation. If it is delayed, learners will tend to discount its relevance. The tutor needs to be a good role model, otherwise feedback will lack credibility.

A conducive learning environment is vital to foster holistic development of students.

The importance of the learning environment

Feedback is not delivered or received in a vacuum. Students will be much more receptive to feedback if the atmosphere is supportive and conducive to learning. One of the main ways to develop a supportive atmosphere is through a long-term educational relationship between tutor and student.[7] Unfortunately, the development of modern curricula in medical schools has often fragmented these relationships. A mentoring system over a prolonged period, which allows mentors to see a student's complete feedback, can enable trust to develop. This can help mentors to safely challenge students' inaccurate self-assessments when necessary (Chapter 27). As FM doctors, we are familiar with the benefits of providing continuity of care.

It is perhaps easy for us to appreciate the benefits of long-term mentoring. In addition to gains for the learners, educators find long-term mentoring a rewarding and worthwhile feature of their role (Chapter 26).

> The communication skills used with patients will help feedback discussions with students.

Reflecting further on our clinical practice helps us appreciate another important barrier to receiving feedback. Strong emotions can be a potent obstacle to patients being open to receive information, especially in consultations that involve receiving bad news. In the same way, students often experience strong emotions when receiving feedback, which can present a significant barrier.[11] This is particularly obvious when they are being told they have failed an assessment or course. It is usually helpful (when possible) to avoid crude pass/fail decisions and instead to concentrate on a more nuanced consideration of strengths and weaknesses. Once the emotions have been appropriately acknowledged and addressed, the learners are normally more receptive to suggestions for further development.[12]

Practical feedback tips

1. Allocate time for observation and feedback and repeat at regular intervals throughout the training period.
2. Involve the learner: What do they want help with?
3. Describe what you saw before giving your interpretation.
4. Vary your style to suit each learner.
5. Use the consultation skills that help you with patients and apply them to the feedback conversation. For example, listen attentively and avoid interrupting. Adopt an open, clarifying, probing question style.
6. Create a supportive atmosphere.
7. Encourage self-assessment and reflection.
8. Remember to show empathy but avoid collusion.
9. Keep it specific. It is often helpful to take detailed quotes of what a student said during an observed consultation, or to give a detailed description of what actually happened.
10. Be brave enough to tackle challenging areas.
11. Be realistic: What can you achieve in one session? Perhaps most importantly: What can the learner cope with?

Conclusion

While feedback may be challenging, it is one of the most rewarding aspects of educational practice. To summarise this chapter in a sentence, we would say: "Treat feedback as a sincere meaningful conversation, not as a formulaic one-way delivery mechanism".

References

1. Van De Ridder JM, Stokking KM, McGaghie WC, Ten Cate OT. What is feedback in clinical education? Med Educ. 2008;42(2):189–97.
2. Ramani S, Könings KD, Ginsburg S, van der Vleuten CP. Twelve tips to promote a feedback culture with a growth mind-set: Swinging the feedback pendulum from recipes to relationships. Med Teach. 2019;41(6):625–31.
3. Dohrenwend A. Serving up the feedback sandwich. Fam Pract Manag. 2002;9(10):43.
4. Kurtz S, Silverman J, Draper J, van Dalen J, Platt FW. Teaching and learning communication skills in medicine. London: CRC Press; 2017.
5. Sargeant J, Armson H, Driessen E, Holmboe E, Könings K, Lockyer J, Lynn L, Mann K, Ross K, Silver I, Soklaridis S. Evidence-informed facilitated feedback: The R2C2 feedback model. MedEdPORTAL. 2016;12. https://www.mededportal.org/doi/epdf/10.15766/mep_2374-8265.10387
6. Boehler ML, Rogers DA, Schwind CJ, Mayforth R, Quin J, Williams RG, Dunnington G. An investigation of medical student reactions to feedback: A randomised controlled trial. Med Educ. 2006;40(8):746–49.
7. Harrison CJ, Könings KD, Dannefer EF, Schuwirth LW, Wass V, van der Vleuten CP. Factors influencing students' receptivity to formative feedback emerging from different assessment cultures. Perspect Med Educ. 2016;5(5):276–84.
8. Lefroy JE, Hawarden A, Gay SP, McKinley RK. Does formal workplace based assessment add value to informal feedback? MedEdPublish. 2017;6(1):27. https://doi.org/10.15694/mep.2017.000027
9. Lefroy J, Watling C, Teunissen PW, Brand P. Guidelines: The do's, don'ts and don't knows of feedback for clinical education. Perspect Med Educ. 2015;4(6):284–99.
10. Harrison CJ. Feedback: The need for meaningful conversations. J Grad Med Educ. 2017;9(2):171.
11. Harrison CJ, Könings KD, Schuwirth L, Wass V, Van der Vleuten C. Barriers to the uptake and use of feedback in the context of summative assessment. Adv Health Sci Educ. 2015;20(1):229–45.
12. Spooner M, Duane C, Uygur J, Smyth E, Marron B, Murphy PJ, Pawlikowska T. Self-regulatory learning theory as a lens on how undergraduate and postgraduate learners respond to feedback: A BEME scoping review: BEME Guide no. 66. Med Teach. 2021;18:1–6.

29

Principles of assessment and assessment tools

Ching-wa Chung and Saniya Sabzwari

SUMMARY OF KEY LEARNING POINTS

- Family medicine (FM) doctors are well placed to develop and deliver assessments for students both within their practices and centrally at the medical school.

- Acquiring supervisory skills to give constructive feedback for formative assessments and to understand competency standards set for summative assessments is important.

- The utility index formula summarises the key principles to use when choosing the tools for assessment and emphasises the importance of ensuring educational impact.

- For FM tutors to be effective role models and credible assessors, they must have the knowledge and familiarity with the tools being used in order to provide assessment that is robust.

- The generalist breadth and diversity of FM practice offers a well-positioned context to provide formative assessments with feedback as an integral part of the curriculum.

- FM placements provide students with multiple assessments given by multiple assessors over time. This offers the best chance of measuring competency in medical education.

Introduction

FM doctors practise in settings that offer a conducive environment for student assessment. Their spectrum of care includes a wide variety of clinical presentations—acute undifferentiated symptoms, multimorbidity, and care of chronic illnesses across all age groups. This provides the opportunity to educate and engage in learner assessment. We strongly encourage FM doctors to add assessment to their educational activities.

DOI: 10.1201/9781003325734-34

Assessment in clinical medicine holds great importance; it tasks the programme and assessors with the responsibility of ensuring the clinical competence of its trainees (Chapter 27). Therefore, FM doctors must invest time and effort in understanding assessment processes and the tools put in place by the educational programme to make crucial decisions on whether students are safe and have reached the standard to progress.

The role of FM doctors

As argued throughout this book, with their broad clinical knowledge, generalist experience, and holistic clinical approach, FM doctors are well-placed to both teach and assess students. The ongoing student contact in their practices, often with 1:1 supervision, provides frequent opportunities to formatively assess *for* learning, i.e. give constructive feedback to build ongoing learning (Chapters 26 and 28). They are also well-placed to develop and deliver summative assessments *of* learning either through workplace-based assessments in their practices or in central school examinations. There are benefits too. Participation in assessment offers clinicians opportunities to stay updated and strengthen their educational portfolios.

> Combining formative skills to deliver assessment *for* learning with competency judgements for summative assessment *of* learning is challenging. FM doctors are well-placed to do both.

Tools for assessment are generally instituted by the medical school curriculum. While the tool is important, it is only as good as its user. Therefore, FM doctors must become familiar with the assessment methods they use, their purpose and implementation. Developing the practice of self-reflection as assessors is crucial to ensure that their assessments have impact.

Key concepts in assessment

To best utilise assessment tools, it is important to be familiar with the factors underpinning the design of an assessment strategy. There are various key principles to consider when doing this. The utility index is a conceptual framework that incorporates these:[1,2]

$$\text{Utility Index} = \text{Reliability} \times \text{Validity} \times \text{Cost} \times \text{Feasibility} \times \text{Educational Impact} \times \text{Acceptability}$$

Reliability relates to how reproducible the results are. That is, if the same assessment was repeated to students of the same standard, how likely are they to score the same?

Validity refers to how accurately the assessment measured the student's ability that is being tested. There are different forms of validity that can be applied.[3]

Cost is clearly an important factor, as is *Feasibility* of delivering the assessment. Feasibility may include resources such as equipment or clinical assessors for medical assessments.

Educational Impact refers to how assessments can drive, or unintendingly influence learning. Students may adapt their learning processes and content to pass assessments. Thus, assessments should be developed with this understanding and carefully selected to robustly align with the learning outcomes. This is called constructive alignment (Chapter 27).

Acceptability, the assessment needs to be acceptable to all involved, students, assessors, regulators, and the public.

Formative and summative assessment

Traditionally, assessment only passed summative judgement on learner performance for progression in an educational programme. Now, assessment has evolved to include support for learners and the learning process. Formative assessment, i.e. assessment *for* learning, measures performance to identify strengths/weaknesses to improve educational outcomes for learners. Summative assessment, i.e. assessment *of* learning, grades performance for pass/fail decisions and student progression.

> Assessment needs careful design to drive learning. It is of paramount importance that the assessment has educational impact and the tools chosen align with the learning outcomes.

Reflective practice and constructive feedback

The practice of reflection as a clinician helps improve our thoughts, interactions, and experiences in practice settings. FM doctors engaged in assessment must extend this reflective practice to their role as assessors. This helps decipher the "hows" and the "whys" of rating performance and understanding individual styles of assessors which are important in quality assurance of assessments (Chapter 19).

Feedback is also essential. Literature highlights that learners feel they get limited feedback opportunities. FM doctors are uniquely placed in their practices to give meaningful 1:1 constructive feedback based on their observations. Such feedback, when given over time, helps improve learner performance (Chapter 28). Pendleton's model provides an effective feedback framework.[4,5]

> For tools to effectively offer assessment "for" learning, reflective practice is essential to help students constructively identify gaps in their learning and set actions plans for further study.

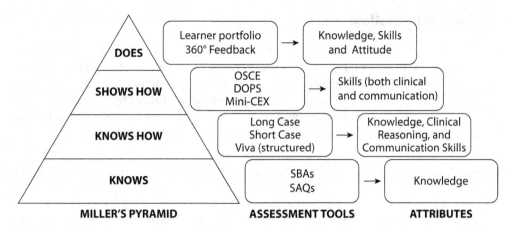

FIGURE 29.1 Miller's pyramid.[5,6]

Levels of competency

When assessing a medical student, one has to consider the competency level that the student is expected to achieve as they progress. Different assessment tools assess different levels of competency. Miller developed a competency framework, known as Miller's pyramid[6,7] (Figure 29.1). He conjectured that students move from the base of the pyramid (knows) before progressing higher (knows how, shows how) until they reach the top (does), as detailed below.

Knowledge, skills, and attitudes

Learning outcomes may relate to knowledge gained, skills learnt, or attitudes adopted. Understanding what you want to assess helps you find the right assessment tools at the appropriate competency level.

Knows

"Knows" refers to acquiring knowledge and information of facts in a particular course of education. This is deemed a prerequisite or a base for further learning which also helps in acquisition of skills and attitudes.

Single best answer multichoice questions

Single best answer (SBA) questions offer a reliable, objective, and valid tool for assessment when broad areas of knowledge need to be tested.[2,8] This involves a question with a single best answer presented within choice of other answers (called distractors). They are cognitively difficult, labour-intensive, and time-consuming to construct and standard set. With their breadth of clinical knowledge, FM doctors are well-placed to construct SBA questions.

Short answer questions

Short answer questions (SAQs), very short answer questions (VSAQs), modified essay questions (MEQs) are all variations on a short question assessment format that requires a short "written" freeform answer (e.g. a clinical vignette followed by a question such as "list the differential diagnoses").[8] They are best accompanied by a marksheet of key responses to ensure minimal examiner subjectivity. Whilst easier to construct, marking SAQs is more labour-intensive and subject to more variation than SBAs.[9]

Knows how

"Knows how" refers to the ability to interpret and apply knowledge. For medical students, this could include the application of clinical reasoning skills to a theoretical case or being able to explain how to conduct a physical examination. If carefully constructed, e.g. by using clinical scenarios where knowledge is applied to reach a diagnosis or management plan, SBAs and SAQs can test at the "knows how" level.

Case-based discussions

These are structured discussions between students and assessors on a clinical case. The discussion includes clinical knowledge, clinical diagnostic reasoning, investigations, and management. For assessment, the discussion can have a structured approach using a variety of proforma templates. As a formative tool, it is very useful to allow students to reflect and identify gaps. For summative assessment, this must be used more carefully as there are many factors that can influence the validity and reliability of CBDs.

Oral examinations/viva: Structured or unstructured

Oral examinations or vivas consist of a student interview by an examiner that can be used to assess application of knowledge and clinical reasoning skills. Subjective assessment, inconsistent marking, and lack of standardisation has reduced its usage and led to the evolution of more structured formats.[10]

Shows how

"Shows how" is the active demonstration of learning by a student.

Mini-clinical evaluation exercise and direct observation of procedural skills

The mini-clinical evaluation exercise (mini-CEX)[11,12] and direct observation of procedural skills (DOPS)[12] both are supervised assessments of student behaviour and actions used to assess clinical competency in the workplace (Chapter 27). For the mini-CEX, a supervisor observes a student undertaking a history and examination in a clinical setting often assessing a differential diagnosis and management plan. DOPS consists of a supervisor observing a student undertaking a clinical procedure in a clinical setting or simulation.

The student and supervisor may agree on a focus for the mini-CEX/DOPS beforehand. The supervisor assesses the performance and provides feedback in a standardised structured format. The mini-CEX/DOPS should ideally be conducted several times by different observers in different contexts. The heterogeneity of patients and presentations in FM are ideal for formative but more challenging for summative assessments (Chapter 27). They may, however, be helpful as part of a portfolio of documented evidence of performance.

Short and long cases

Short cases consist of a small number (usually up to six) of quick clinical cases, with real patients. The student is taken around by the examiner and asked to examine specific systems, elicit clinical signs, and give differential diagnoses.

Long cases[13] are longer (up to an hour) where students are often expected to undertake a full history and examination unsupervised or supervised. This will be followed by a discussion with an examiner.

Both suffer from significant reliability issues. There is no standardisation of questioning by examiners, nor calibration of expectations. These disadvantages led to the development of the objective structured long-case examination record (OSLER) which helps address some of these disadvantages[13].

Objective structured clinical examinations

The objective structured clinical examination (OSCE) is widely used to assess clinical competence and skills.[14,15] It consists of students moving through a sequence of clinical cases or "stations". Stations are designed to assess the student's performance on specific clinical tasks such as taking a history or clinical examination. Each student has the same standardised assessment. This includes the same stations, completing the same tasks, using standardised simulated or real patients, marked by a standardised structured marking scheme. Marking is against a checklist or rating scales. The station duration varies, but is usually 5–15 minutes. The number of stations varies with reliability improving progressively as stations increase but organisation becoming more challenging. These features make OSCEs well-suited to high stakes clinical assessments. However, OSCEs are very complex to set up, require detailed planning, some expertise, and are very resource-intensive to run.[15]

FM doctors are qualified to assess diverse clinical presentations. They should be encouraged to participate in question setting in the context of primary care and to attend as OSCE examiners where the presence of the FM faculty is important.

FM doctors should be actively involved within the medical school in writing questions in primary care contexts, setting standards, and being trained to attend as summative OSCE examiners.

Does

"Does" relates to what the student/future doctor actually does in clinical practice. What is their actual and unobserved behaviour? This is challenging to assess, but some tools that can help are outlined below. However, it needs to be acknowledged that when observed, actual behaviour can change.

Direct observation

FM doctors must include direct and ongoing observation to assess learners. While most educational programmes struggle with obtaining a satisfactory number of direct observations, FM doctors have the advantage of frequent student contact in a clinical practice setting where patients seek ongoing care making direct observation of learners more feasible. This can include the mini-CEX and DOPS as previously outlined.

Supervisor's report

A supervisor's report is a statement by the educational supervisor of the student's progress and performance often at the end of a clinical attachment. This can have varied formats but may include assessment of clinical knowledge, clinical skills, clinical reasoning, clinical management, communication skills, team working, and rapport with patients. FM placements with low student-to-supervisor ratio, high personal student contact, and the involvement of a wide primary care team are particularly well-placed to make such assessments. However, this closer relationship may result in a reluctance to report poor performance (Chapter 26).

360-Degree (multi-source) feedback

Feedback from different members of the multidisciplinary team, and even patients, can be sought. This is best done anonymously and using formal mechanisms, but can be informal and individual. However, these do not provide direct observations but rely on the individual's recall and perceptions of a student's behaviour. This tool is more often used in postgraduate rather than undergraduate medical education.[16]

The generalist breadth of FM practice, diversity of patient presentations, and close supervision are ideal for assessing students formatively on their performance and attitudinal behaviours.

Portfolios

A portfolio is a collection of evidence that demonstrates achieving competencies or outcomes often supported by reflection on performance and learning plans. It may be unstructured, or have very specific requirements (e.g. a set number of mini-CEXs and DOPs). A portfolio can be used to evidence knowledge and skills, attitude, and professionalism. It is important to be clear about the aim of the portfolio as this influences the design of the portfolio.

In FM, the opportunity to collect evidence for a portfolio is plentiful, such as mini-CEX, DOPS, CBD, reflective accounts, peer or team feedback, and even patient feedback. FM doctors should make themselves familiar with any requirements for students' portfolios and support the student in collating the evidence.[17]

Barriers to involving FM doctors in assessment

FM doctors do encounter challenges. It is important to acknowledge and understand these to stay academically engaged. The biggest barriers are time constraints and clinical commitments. Some FM doctors hesitate to take on the additional responsibility of education in busy clinics. Lack of confidence in teaching ability is another barrier that prevents FM doctors from engaging in teaching and assessment.

Some learners may be less comfortable with more remote clinical practices. Others may feel the best learning takes place in in-patient and hospital settings rather than in family practice. While patient care always takes precedence, dedicating one day a week to teaching with a limited number of students may be a reasonable option for a busy practitioner. It is important, given the priority students place on assessment, that FM tutors are seen to actively engage in both formative and summative tests.

> Given the importance students place on assessments, FM tutors must be active both formatively and summatively to ensure FM is perceived as important and not marginalised.

Attending educational workshops and conferences can help familiarise FM doctors with basic teaching and assessment skills, boosting confidence and comfort during both. FM doctors placed in remote sites may choose to tutor on occasion at sites other than their own to help increase engagement with learners. For some, clinical teaching may not be remunerated; however, the rewards of engaging in education lie in one's own professional growth, keeping up to date with current knowledge and practice and the personal satisfaction and joy in teaching.

Conclusion

FM doctors can play a vital role in the assessment of medical students. The FM setting allows valuable and unique opportunities to assess students during clinical attachments. In addition, FM doctors' generalist clinical knowledge and skills make them valuable assets in delivering assessments within a medical school. It is important for FM doctors to be familiar and competent in delivering these assessments.

References

1. Van Der Vleuten CPM, Schuwirth LWT. Assessing professional competence: From methods to programmes. Med Educ. 2005;39(3):309–17.
2. Mirbahai LW, Adie J. Applying the utility index to review single best answer questions in medical education assessment. Arch Epidemiol Public Heal. 2020;2(1). doi: 10.15761/AEPH.1000113
3. Colliver JA, Conlee MJ, Verhulst SJ. From test validity to construct validity... and back? Med Educ. 2012;46(4):366–71.
4. Pendleton D, Schofield T, Tate P. The consultation: An approach to learning and teaching. Oxford: Oxford University Press; 1984. pp. 68–71.
5. Burgess A, van Diggele C, Roberts C, Mellis C. Feedback in the clinical setting. BMC Med Educ [Internet]. 2020;20(Suppl. 2):1–5. Available from: http://dx.doi.org/10.1186/s12909-020-02280-5
6. Miller GE. The assessment of clinical skills/competence/performance. Acad Med. 1990;65(9):S63–S67.
7. Witheridge A, Ferns G, Scott-Smith W. Revisiting Miller's pyramid in medical education: The gap between traditional assessment and diagnostic reasoning. Int J Med Educ. 2019;10:191–92.
8. Webber RH. Structured short-answer questions: An alternative examination method. Med Educ. 1992;26(1):58–62.
9. Sam AH, Westacott R, Gurnell M, Wilson R, Meeran K, Brown C. Comparing single-best-answer and very-short-answer questions for the assessment of applied medical knowledge in 20 UK medical schools: Cross-sectional study. BMJ Open. 2019;9(9):e032550.
10. Anbarasi K, Karunakaran J, Ravichandran L, Arthi B. Effectiveness of the structured and conventional methods of viva examination in medical education: A systematic review and meta-analysis. J Clin Diagnostic Res. 2022;16(9):1–7.
11. Norcini JJ, Blank LL, Duffy FD, Fortna GS. The mini-CEX: A method for assessing clinical skills. Ann Intern Med. 2003;138(6):476–81.
12. Norcini J, Burch V. Workplace-based assessment as an educational tool: AMEE Guide no. 31. Med Teach. 2007;29(9–10):855–71.
13. Ponnamperuma GG, Karunathilake IM, McAleer S, Davis MH. The long case and its modifications: A literature review. Med Educ. 2009;43(10):936–41.
14. Khan KZ, Ramachandran S, Gaunt K, Pushkar P. The objective structured clinical examination (OSCE): AMEE guide no. 81. Part I: An historical and theoretical perspective. Med Teach. 2013;35(9):e1437–e46.
15. Khan KZ, Gaunt K, Ramachandran S, Pushkar P. The objective structured clinical examination (OSCE): AMEE Guide no. 81. Part II: Organisation & administration. Med Teach. 2013;2(35):1447–63.
16. Donnon T, Al Ansari A, Al Alawi S, Violato C. The reliability, validity, and feasibility of multisource feedback physician assessment: A systematic review. Acad Med. 2014;89:511–6.
17. Van Tartwijk J, Driessen EW. Portfolios for assessment and learning: AMEE Guide no. 45. Med Teach. 2009;31(9):790–801.

30

Struggling students and fitness to practise

Allyn Walsh and Zorayda Leopando

SUMMARY OF KEY LEARNING POINTS

- Medical students almost always hold good academic records. It needs to be recognised that even high-achieving students can struggle during medical school.
- The reasons for student difficulties are usually multifactorial. Often interventions at multiple levels, including addressing external factors, are required.
- Thorough assessment is critical taking student, tutor, and programme perspectives of underlying factors, including knowledge, skills, professionalism, and personal health.
- Remediation efforts should be focused on the root causes of the problems. The educational system and teachers may be contributing to student difficulties.
- Students requiring formal intervention need structured remediation with honest, supportive tutors trained to challenge students' ideas and approaches to learning.
- Transparent, fair, defensible school policies and procedures are essential when, rarely, remediation fails and students need to be dismissed from the programme.
- Family medicine (FM) doctors, given their skills in taking a holistic approach to complex multifactorial problems, are well-placed to support struggling students.

The importance of assisting struggling medical students

Medical students tend to be highly motivated to become excellent physicians. While the competitiveness of entry to medical schools varies widely between countries, many students when admitted have a track record of academic success. Despite this, there is a subset of medical students who have significant difficulties during the course. These difficulties may include knowledge and skills deficits, maladaptive behaviour, as well as personal and health issues. Often these problems coexist and must be considered together.

DOI: 10.1201/9781003325734-35

Most institutions and stake holders have invested heavily in producing physicians. Attrition is thus costly. Furthermore, teachers can find dealing with students in difficulty challenging and discouraging.[1-3] It is not only imperative for students' sakes to identify and remediate difficulties. It is important for faculty members, the educational institution, the healthcare system, and, of course, for patients and the community that medical students are supported to reach their potential.

The multifaceted nature of medical student struggles

Case example Part 1: Joe

Joe is preparing to enter the clinical years of medical school training. While he initially did quite well, his grades have gradually slipped. He risks failing to progress to the next clinical level. One tutor complained that Joe is lazy and should be removed from the programme. What could be going wrong? It is simple to think that he is not putting the required effort into his study. This may be a significant factor. But Joe's situation needs considering more broadly: not only WHAT he has achieved or failed to achieve, but also WHY this is happening.

There are many possible factors contributing to a student's struggles. When difficulties are serious and profound, interventions at multiple levels can bring seemingly challenging, or even insurmountable, problems down to a manageable size. Factors external to the student can contribute significantly and may also need addressing.

When a medical student is having significant difficulty in the programme, there is usually more than one underlying factor. As in patient care, a thorough assessment is necessary.

To discuss medical student problems and deficits, we have divided the issues into three interacting categories: (i) knowledge and skills; (ii) professionalism and behaviour; and (iii) personal and health issues and applied these separately to the roles of students, teachers, and the education programmes. Table 30.1 summarises these.

Knowledge and skill deficits

Medical students may struggle with absorbing and applying large amounts of information, have difficulty with effective time management, or have inadequate study strategies.[4] To become a physician, good self-regulated learning is essential. A cycle of internal goal setting, taking action to fulfil the goals, self-monitoring of achievement, and, finally, reflection and planning for next steps is fundamental (Chapter 19).

TABLE 30.1 The struggling medical student: Potential contributing factors

	Knowledge and skill	Professional behaviour*/ attitude	Personal/health
Student	• Poor study/learning skills • Difficulty applying knowledge to practice • Poor problem-solving or clinical reasoning skills • Poor time management or organisational skills • Difficulty with case/clinical presentations • Poor communication and/or relationship skills • Poor manual skills	• Poor professional responsibility • Attendance problems/ lateness • "Boundary" concerns • Defensive with feedback and coaching • Disrespectful behaviour • Dishonesty • Poor work habits or lack effort • Assignments not done	• Mental health problems • Substance abuse • Physical health problems or limitations • Learning disabilities • Personal issues—family health problems, child or elder care, partner issues, sexual orientation issues, etc. • Financial pressures • Transportation issues
Teacher	• Lacks knowledge of objectives • Unrealistic expectations for stage of learner • Expectations/objectives not agreed • Poor feedback and coaching skills • Lacks knowledge of assessment • Inexperience/lack confidence in own skills	• Problematic reactions: • Avoiding the student • Being angry/defensive • Overcommitted to "save" the student • Not approachable or available to student • Inflexible / unwilling to address student needs	• Health or personal problems affecting: • Expectations, • Reactions • Availability to students
Education programme	• Expectations and objectives not clear • Expectations unrealistic • Inadequate teaching and learning resources • Poor communication or lack of agreement between teachers	• Excessive workload • Scheduling problems— inflexibility or inadequate notice • Unwillingness to accommodate learner needs • "Culture" of abuse, intimidation, and/or discrimination	• Resources unavailable to support and address student health or personal needs

Source: Modified from the Programme for Faculty Development, McMaster University, Canada.

*Behaviour to patients, peers, staff.

It has been shown that some struggling students have difficulty with this process.[5] This impairs learning. Fostering an individual medical trainee's self-regulatory beliefs and behaviours may be helpful.[6]

> Reflexivity and self-regulation are key to achieving the lifelong learning skills physicians need. Struggling students may need support in their self-regulatory beliefs and behaviours.

Deficiencies in knowledge and skills can also lie with tutors. Teachers may not understand the learning outcomes set for students or have realistic expectations of their abilities. Failure to understand assessment processes can impede identifying student difficulties. Poor feedback and coaching may impair students' abilities to grow their knowledge and skills.

Lastly, the educational programme may be contributing to student struggles. The teaching resources may be inadequate to meet student needs, learning expectations and outcomes may be poorly established, and communication between the programme and those providing and receiving it may be lacking.

Advising struggling students simply to "read or study more" is unlikely to correct problems in this area. *Remediation*, rather than *repetition*, is required.[7,8] To understand where the problems lie, students must feel safe to disclose their difficulties and describe their study and learning processes.

> Simply advising struggling students to "read or study more" is unlikely to help correct problems. Remediation in a safe environment rather than repetition is required.

An appropriate remediation system needs to be established for students whose difficulties require formal intervention. Remediation requires honest, supportive facilitators who can challenge students' ideas and approaches to learning. To "diagnose" problems and guide necessary changes, a good understanding of how people learn is essential. Rather than re-teaching content, a remediation tutor helps struggling students become independent learners.[4] This is not a role for every tutor.

Identifying teachers' learning needs is essential. Faculty development (teacher training) to ensure solid skills in feedback, assessment, and coaching should be available to all tutors (Chapter 26). Finally, educational programmes need to periodically evaluate the established programme learning outcomes and expectations, revise them as appropriate, and ensure adequate sustainable resourcing (Chapter 31).

Institutions and educational programmes experience great variability in their funding which impacts on resourcing student remediation. Some well-resourced programmes can provide a formal structure. However, for most educational programmes, relatively simple measures should be possible by providing students access to a mentor or advisor, and/or training tutors to deal with students in difficulty. It is important that students have somewhere to go for help.

> Relatively simple measures such as providing students access to mentors and training tutors to deal with students in difficulty should be possible even in low-resource programmes.

Professionalism and behavioural deficits

Struggles with professional behaviour are often perceived as very challenging and may evoke considerable emotion amongst students and teachers. Chapter 12 discusses integrating professionalism positively within the curriculum. Here we will discuss individual student difficulties with professional behaviour. Problems may include attendance, punctuality, and lack of responsibility. Defensiveness with feedback and coaching can hinder student development and cause interpersonal difficulties. There may be disrespectful behaviour to patients, peers, and staff and even outright dishonesty. Teachers may develop problematic reactions to students, such as avoidance or anger. Unavailable, unapproachable, and inflexible tutors can aggravate student issues.

Educational programmes without clear and well-disseminated policies on standards of behaviour miss an important tool for identifying and remediating professionalism issues. Some programmes may demand excessive student workloads. Teachers may be inflexible and unable to accommodate learning needs. At the extreme, educational programmes may tolerate a culture of abuse, intimidation, and/or discrimination.

The information-gathering process is more difficult when examining behavioural difficulties than for knowledge and skills, where routine and consistent assessments are commonly the norm. As with any complex problem, hearing from the student as well as teachers and programme staff is important to gain a thorough understanding. Students will again benefit from discussions with a trusted, honest mentor. Agreeing clear expectations of behaviour with regular reviews of progress is helpful.

> Professional behaviour deficits can incite difficult emotions between students and teachers and be challenging. Clear faculty guidelines on handling these issues are essential.

Rarely, transgressions are severe enough and progress on change so inadequate that students may have to leave the programme. While there is insufficient evidence to make absolute statements on best remediation practice for addressing professionalism issues,[9] it is essential that programme support and guidance to teachers is clearly outlined to help them deal with this difficult area.[10]

A discussion of professionalism issues amongst teachers and programmes is beyond this chapter's limits, but it is important to recognise the impact of teacher behaviour on students, which can affect learning and well-being. Tolerance by institutions of intimidation and abuse is unacceptable (Chapter 25).

Personal and health issues

When students are struggling, it is important to look beyond their exam achievements and behaviour to explore personal or health issues. All too often students will not admit to problems, either physical or mental, because of concerns about stigma and impact on their career. A myriad of health issues such as physical limitations, learning disabilities, and mental health problems may impact student learning and behaviour. Severe financial stress, family problems, and other social issues can affect their performance.[11] These problems need to be identified and ameliorated for students to thrive in medical school.

Teachers may face similar challenges and require support. Educational programmes can help by facilitating healthcare availability for students and staff and finding ways to provide students with financial aid or support. An advisor system may offer students a trusted confident who can direct them to help.[12]

Case example Part 2: Joe

Joe may not be spending sufficient time studying. Why would this be? He could be disinterested/unmotivated. His learning could be impaired by personal issues such as family, relationship, or health issues. His strategy for academic success in secondary school may be inappropriate for the self-regulated learning required in medical school. His teachers may lack solid knowledge of learning outcomes or expected competency at his current clinical level or have missed training on assessment processes, feedback, or coaching.

Although Joe's medical school assigned an advisor to every student, he has been avoiding meeting his. When she eventually does manage to meet him, they established a good relationship. He became confident she wanted him to succeed. Further discussion revealed that he initially felt overwhelmed with the volume of material he needed to learn. He had recently joined a peer study group and recognised that his approach of taking and memorising voluminous notes was inappropriate. He now set personal learning outcomes before every session and felt this would help in time. His greater problem though was financial. To support his family and himself, Joe was working long hours in a restaurant. He lacked sleep, was anxious, felt very stressed, and was ashamed he had avoided his advisor. He was unaware of the medical school bursary programme until his advisor directed him to apply. She recommended he continue the study group meetings. Personally, she then sought training on coaching effective learning strategies.

Multifaceted approach

As stated above, when dealing with struggling students, there is usually more than one underlying factor. As in patient care, a thorough assessment is necessary before management strategies are established. Progress is more easily made in the context of a trusted relationship. FM teachers, given their generalist holistic approach to patients and skills in dealing with complex undifferentiated clinical presentations, are well-placed to train as remediation tutors within medical schools.

Remediation interventions should be targeted to specific difficulties. Rarely is one intervention adequate. Regular reassessment to gauge progress is intrinsic to eventual student success.[13] Resources vary hugely globally but thinking broadly about the factors impairing progress for struggling students can help identify appropriate interventions within available resources.

> Remediation should include interventions targeted to the student's specific difficulties. Regular reassessment to gauge progress is important for eventual student success.

When remediation is insufficient

Unfortunately, despite efforts, duty to society, patients, and the profession can occasionally require educational programmes to dismiss students. Barriers to failing underperforming trainees have been identified.[1–3] These include lack of documentation, fear of repercussions, including legal actions and appeals, and lack of support and resources for staff. Concern for the student can make tutors reluctant to confront them, particularly if they perceive a lack of known remediation options.

Globally there is huge variability between institutional culture and legal requirements. Detailed guidance on removing students from the programme is difficult. Suffice it to say that to reach this stage, the educational programme must have a strong and defensible assessment programme and have made clear efforts to support and remediate the student. Performance standards for academic achievement and professional behaviour must be clearly outlined. Institutional support for staff and support from colleagues can help make these difficult decisions.[3] Table 30.2 outlines the requirements for a robust and fair system for these situations.

> To dismiss a student, the educational programme must have a strong and defensible assessment programme and have made clear efforts to support and remediate the student.

TABLE 30.2 Institutional requirements for dealing with struggling students

- Transparent educational objectives, expectations, and standards
- Robust student assessment programme, including a variety of reliable and valid tools
- Remediation opportunities for students (and teachers) with regular reassessment
- Fair and transparent dismissal and appeals processes
- Strong faculty development on student assessment with documentation of progress
- Support and guidance for teachers and students involved in remediation and dismissal processes

Conclusion

When students are struggling to succeed in their programme, it is important to assess their situation broadly and consider how teachers and the educational programme may assist them or conversely may be hindering their progress. Remediation is easier and more likely to succeed if an individualised approach is taken which identifies and addresses the root causes. While most remediation is likely to be successful, it is important that the educational programme has a robust and fair system for handling failures that may lead to student dismissal. Facilitating the success of medical students is important for not just the individual student, but also for their teachers, their institution, and the community. FM doctors should be encouraged to take part in remediation processes; seeing students begin to flourish and achieve is one of the most satisfying aspects of being a medical teacher.

References

1. Dudek NL, Marks MB, Regehr G. Failure to fail: The perspectives of clinical supervisors. Acad Med. 2005;80(10):S84–S7.
2. Guraya SY, van Mook WN, Khoshhal KI. Failure of faculty to fail failing medical students: Fiction or an actual erosion of professional standards? J Taibah Univ Med Sci. 2019;14(2):103.
3. Yepes-Rios M, Dudek N, Duboyce R, Curtis J, Allard RJ, Varpio L. The failure to fail underperforming trainees in health professions education: A BEME systematic review: BEME Guide no. 42. Med Teach. 2016;38(11):1092–99.
4. Winston KA, Van Der Vleuten CP, Scherpbier AJ. The role of the teacher in remediating at-risk medical students. Med Teach. 2012;34(11):e732–e42.
5. Patel R, Tarrant C, Bonas S, Yates J, Sandars J. The struggling student: A thematic analysis from the self-regulated learning perspective. Med Educ. 2015;49(4):417–26.
6. Durning SJ, Cleary TJ, Sandars J, Hemmer P, Kokotailo P, Artino AR. Perspective: Viewing "strugglers" through a different lens: How a self-regulated learning perspective can help medical educators with assessment and remediation. Acad Med. 2011;86(4):488–95.
7. Cleland J, Leggett H, Sandars J, Costa MJ, Patel R, Moffat M. The remediation challenge: Theoretical and methodological insights from a systematic review. Med Educ. 2013;47(3):242–51.
8. Audetat Voirol MC, Laurin S, Dory V. Remediation for struggling learners: Putting an end to 'more of the same'. Med Educ. 2013;47(3):230–31.
9. Brennan N, Price T, Archer J, Brett J. Remediating professionalism lapses in medical students and doctors: A systematic review. Med Educ. 2020;54(3):196–204.
10. Rougas S, Gentilesco B, Green E, Flores L. Twelve tips for addressing medical student and resident physician lapses in professionalism. Med Teach. 2015;37(10):901–7.
11. Aziz A, Mahboob U, Sethi A. What problems make students struggle during their undergraduate medical education? A qualitative exploratory study. Pak J Med Sci. 2020;36(5):1020.
12. Swan Sein A, Daniel M, Fleming A, Morrison G, Christner JG, Esposito K, Pock AR, Grochowski CO, Dalrymple JL, Santen SA. Identifying and supporting students to prevent USMLE step 1 failures when testing follows clerkships: Insights from 9 schools. Acad Med. 2020;95(9):1338–45.
13. Ridinger H, Cvengros J, Gunn J, Tanaka P, Rencic J, Tekian A, Park YS. Struggling medical learners: A competency-based approach to improving performance. MedEdPORTAL. 2018;14:10739.

Evaluating teaching and learning across the curriculum

We do not receive wisdom. We must discover it for ourselves after experience which no one else can have for us and from which no one can spare us.

Marcel Proust

31

Quality improvement and evaluation

Esther M. Johnston and Akye Essuman

SUMMARY OF KEY LEARNING POINTS

- Evaluation and quality improvement (QI) are complementary, sometimes overlapping, processes that must be embedded in undergraduate family medicine (FM) training throughout the programme.
- Programmes should define their target outcomes, guided by institutional, regional, and national/international standards, to identify success in these areas.
- Measurable performance indicators and attainable time-bound targets should be defined across three domains: academic, the learning environment, and long-term outcomes.
- When evaluation identifies opportunities for growth, established approaches such as the plan-do-study-act (PDSA) or context-input-process-product (CIPP) are useful models for QI.
- Evaluation processes can be used as advocacy tools to demonstrate the value of FM clerkships both within the undergraduate medical curriculum and even globally on workforce development.

Principles of programme evaluation and quality improvement

Programme evaluation (PE) is the process of assessing an educational programme's design, implementation, and outcomes in comparison to accepted standards or agreed-upon benchmarks. QI is a complementary, often overlapping, process in which efforts are undertaken to recalibrate the training programme to bring aspects of the programme closer to meeting the previously identified standards.

The primary purpose of PE/QI is to gain information about a programme's performance and value, and make recommendations for achieving improvement

DOI: 10.1201/9781003325734-37

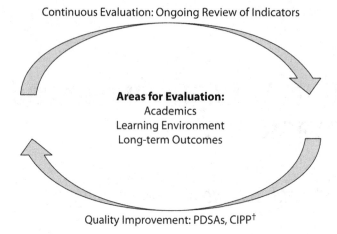

Continuous Evaluation: Ongoing Review of Indicators

Areas for Evaluation:
Academics
Learning Environment
Long-term Outcomes

Quality Improvement: PDSAs, CIPP†

†PDSA: Plan-Do-Study-Act; CIPP: Context-Input-Process-Product

FIGURE 31.1 Cyclic process of programme evaluation and quality improvement.

where indicated. PE and QI are valuable, reciprocal processes for educators and training programme leaders as they work to strengthen the quality of the education. To achieve maximum impact, they should be routine, continuous processes, in which data is generated through evaluation. Systematic regular assessment of the evaluation data then feeds into QI processes[1,2] (Figure 31.1).

PE/QI has key benefits for the student, educator, programme leadership, the educational institution, and, ultimately, patients:

- *Students* are empowered to improve the programme for current and future colleagues. Through the evaluation process, they can give feedback on their experiences of curriculum content and the learning environment. Evaluation data, and the resulting QI initiatives, drive modifications and updates of programme content and delivery methods. This ensures the curriculum remains relevant to learner needs.

- *Educators* receive positive reinforcement on their efforts and feedback on areas for improvement to further their own professional development. In addition, they potentially receive support in achieving those improvements.

- *Programme leadership* receives information on the needs, challenges, and expectations of students on content, delivery methods, and the overall learning environment. This enables programme leaders to determine if the programme is achieving its intended learning outcomes over time. QI processes enable programme leadership to improve for the future.

- *Institutions* benefit as PE/QI provides accountability. Regular evaluation facilitates the production of reports on programme effectiveness. These may be required for review by the university or college administration to inform decisions on whether to continue, postpone, or cancel a programme.

Evaluation data and evidence of QI processes may be required for accreditation by regional and national regulatory bodies, and for support from funding agencies.

■ *Patients and society* ultimately benefit as PE/QI processes ensure that educational programmes disseminate and provide training and update on the most current medical knowledge and practices.

> PE and QI are continuous practices in which processes are reviewed and adjusted to achieve expected outcomes and meet changing standards in educational programmes, including undergraduate FM.

Conducting programme evaluation

Periodic evaluation of programme quality should be comprehensive, assessing all programme domains and functions. It should reflect the goals and values of the individual training site, and any regional, national, or specialty-specific accrediting bodies.[3,4]

While specifics may vary from one training programme to another, there are some programme domains which are applicable to almost all training sites. These include the programme's ability to meet the needs of the following:

i. *Academics:* The programme's effectiveness at ensuring students gain medical knowledge and clinical skills, and, in FM, skills in coordinating community-oriented primary care.

ii. *The learning environment:* The programme's ability to ensure a safe and well-resourced setting for trainees, with high-quality teachers and supervision.

iii. *Long-term outcomes:* The programme's ability to leave a positive impression on trainees of FM as a discipline.[3]

When performing evaluations to determine if success is being met in each domain, it is critical to identify specific, measurable indicators and attainable, realistic, time-bound targets. Table 31.1 provides examples of evaluation indicators for each domain—academic, learning environment, and long-term outcomes.

Additionally, it is recommended that programmes evaluate, with some regularity, the evaluation tools themselves that are being utilised to assess the above three domains. The mechanisms for doing this may vary from site to site. For example: (i) A faculty member may be assigned to perform a literature review of new assessment methodologies for evaluating clinical skills. (ii) A course chair may review the class performance on an exam and consider whether certain questions should be written more clearly to better assess medical knowledge. (iii) The department faculty and student representative may meet as a group periodically to discuss if a

TABLE 31.1 Monitoring and evaluation framework

Domains for programme evaluation		Example indicators
Academic	Medical knowledge	• Student performance on interim assessments of exams and achievement
	Clinical skills	• Student performance on standardised workplace-based clinical skills tests
	Ability to engage in community-oriented partnership/primary care	• Student completion and performance on community-oriented primary care projects
Learning environment	Safety and support of learners	• Student satisfaction with learner-oriented approach on evaluations of faculty
		• Spot assessments of personal protective equipment in clinical learning spaces
	Resources for effective teaching and learning	• Learner satisfaction with accessibility of electronic course website or resources
		• Availability of key journals or texts from which required readings are assigned
	Faculty knowledge/quality	• Level of faculty engagement in department-recommended continuing medical education
Long-term outcomes	Student interest in FM	• Number of undergraduate FM students who elect to enter FM as a specialty
		• Change in student numbers interested in a FM career pre- and post-rotation

learner survey is adequately collecting key information about the training environment.

> FM undergraduate training programmes should regularly assess the quality of evaluation methods used to assess academic content, the learning environment, and the ability to improve student interest.

We offer examples of evaluation in action:

Example 1

Evaluation of academics: The City FM Department requires all undergraduate students rotating through their FM rotation to sit a national standardised exam at the end of the rotation. The department uses the percentage of students passing this exam as an indicator of the programme's academic quality. It sets a target of at least 98% student passing on the first try in a given academic year. The department checks this indicator yearly to ensure its goal is met. If it falls short of 98%, it uses a standardised QI process to identify and address any factors leading to this lapse.

Example 2

Evaluation of learning environments: The National University FM Department places medical students with FM tutors at clinics and hospitals dispersed across the country. On completing every clinical rotation, students fill in an anonymous evaluation rating, using a Likert scale, of their training sites in several areas (e.g. personal protective equipment (PPE) availability, personal safety at the clinical site, supportiveness of the clinical tutor). At the middle and end of every academic year, the department aggregates and looks at these evaluations to assess the safety and quality of the learning environment. Midway through one academic year, they note that one site has consistently poor student scores for PPE accessibility. It initiates an investigation using a standard QI process to identify and address the lapse in PPE availability and then follows the evaluation scores to ensure that the situation has improved.

Mechanisms for quality improvement

QI is a reciprocal process to evaluation. Sometimes the two processes may overlap. Through evaluation (as in the examples shown), deficiencies can be identified. These gaps are then addressed through standardised QI processes. Many different QI processes exist for use in healthcare. A variety of these models has been applied to conduct PE/QI within educational programmes.[5–9] Two of the most used models are as follows:

- *CIPP:* A model in which comprehensive information about the larger context in which the programme operates, and the resources with which it does so, is collected. This may then be used to help develop strategies to respond to identified gaps and improve programme effectiveness or plan for the future of a programme.[7–10]

Example 3

QI/CIPP—Faculty knowledge: The City FM Department offers continuing education and training for tutors who teach undergraduate students in community clinics and hospitals. *Context:* The department conducts regular evaluations of tutors and students, and this year recognises a trend in the need for increased tutor training on how to provide student feedback. *Input:* The department identifies a faculty member with expertise in feedback models to chair a day-long retreat for tutors on this topic and budgets accordingly. *Process:* The faculty chair conducts the retreat and arranges for pre- and post-evaluation to assess improvements in tutor knowledge and workshop satisfaction. *Product:* The department monitors in following months its evaluations of tutors and students to assess if the event resulted in improvements in frequency of feedback received and tutor confidence in delivering feedback.

- *PDSA:* The PDSA is a rapid cycle improvement process which can be used iteratively to assess whether a given change or series of changes leads to a desired outcome/improvement.[11]

Example 4

QI PDSA—academics: The Regional College FM Department identifies through student evaluation that many wanted better training on obtaining patient histories on non-prescription and/or recreational drug use. They decide to conduct a PDSA on a new didactic teaching module. *Plan:* A faculty member, with expertise in this area, designs a lecture-based teaching session. An anonymous pre- and post-survey to evaluate their confidence and knowledge on this history-taking is created to give students before and after the workshop. The goal is to improve baseline confidence and knowledge by at least 30%. *DO:* At the workshop, students complete the pre- and post-surveys. *STUDY:* Faculty then evaluate the survey data. The students demonstrate 85% improvement in knowledge, but only 25% in confidence. *ACT:* The department adopts the workshop into the didactic curriculum but adapts it to include more simulation and practice time to better build student confidence in these history-taking skills. For the next student cohort on the FM rotation, the PDSA cycle is repeated with the improved workshop. The department repeats and acts on the evaluation.

While it is important to choose an effective QI model to guide one's efforts, it is also essential that the programme selects a QI process that fits within its capacity to maintain and implement it regularly.

> Evaluation and QI processes must be selected which are feasible and sustainable for the department to conduct routinely and continuously and can be utilised to inform and improve the programme.

Programme evaluation as a tool to ensure effective placement of FM in the undergraduate curriculum

FM clerkships offer unique opportunities to teach community-oriented primary care and clinical skills. Early student exposure to FM through these clerkships can increase student interest in pursuing it as a career (Chapter 15). Evaluation processes to capture these impacts are thus an important advocacy tool to demonstrate the positive impacts of including FM clerkships within the undergraduate curriculum, demonstrating not just how the undergraduate FM course may positively impact clinical skills and knowledge, but improved interest in primary care careers as well.

In 2018, the global community committed to the Declaration of Astana, re-emphasising its earlier commitments to the 1978 Alma Ata Declaration to invest in health systems that value and prioritise primary healthcare as the means to ensure universal health coverage.[12,13] To meet this goal, national government signatories committed to investing in the training of healthcare professionals able to provide effective primary care, priorities which have been communicated to many national health professional training institutions. Globally, FM educators have used evaluation to demonstrate FM's critical place in the undergraduate medical curriculum. Utilising student evaluation to show improved interest in pursuing careers in community-based primary care as a result of their clerkship exposure has proved invaluable.[14,15] This is just one example of how PE may be used as an advocacy tool to highlight the value of FM clerkship exposure to meet the larger goals of the undergraduate curriculum, health professional training institutions, and even national health system priorities.

Conclusion

PE and QI are two complementary, continuous, and at times intersecting, processes. Routine evaluation should assess the programme's academics, the quality of the learning environment, long-term outcomes, and, ultimately, the evaluation processes themselves. However, PE alone does not result in meaningful change or improvements. It is the role of QI processes to address the findings uncovered through evaluation. There are many PE tools and QI models to act on the outcomes arising from PE, but ultimately the best system is the one that the programme is able to utilise regularly and sustain. Ultimately, ensuring practical, regular, sustainable, and effective processes for PE/QI in undergraduate FM education training programme is essential to ensure that educational programmes remain responsive to the needs of learners and teachers, accountable to institutional and accrediting bodies, and relevant to and representative of the current state of medical knowledge and practice.

References

1. Wong BM, Headrick LA. Application of continuous quality improvement to medical education. Med Educ. 2021;55:72–81.
2. Stalmeijer RE, Whittingham JRD, Bendermacher GWG, Wolfhagen IHAP, Dolmans DHJM, Sehlbach C. Continuous enhancement of educational quality: Fostering a quality culture—AMEE guide. Med Teach. 2023;45(1):6–16.
3. Yale Poorvu Centre for Teaching and Learning. Programme evaluation. Available from: https://poorvucenter.yale.edu/Program-Evaluation
4. Barzansky B, Hunt D, Moineau G, Duckson A, Chi-Wan L, Humphrey H, Peterson L. Continuous quality improvement in an accreditation system for undergraduate medical education: Benefits and challenges. Med Teach. 2015;37:1032–38.
5. Institute for Healthcare Improvement. Quality improvement essentials toolkit. Available from: http://www.ihi.org/resources/Pages/Tools/Quality-Improvement-Essentials-Toolkit.aspx

6. Gibson K, Boyle P, Black DA, Cunningham M, Grimm MC, McNeil HP. Enhancing evaluation in an undergraduate medical education programme. Acad Med. 2008;83:787–93.

7. Yale Poorvu Centre for Teaching and Learning. CIPP model. Available from: https://poorvucenter.yale.edu/CIPP

8. Kulasegaram K, Mylopoulos M, Tonin P, Bernstein S, Bryden P, Law M, Lazor J, Pittini R, Sockalingam S, Tait G, Houston P. The alignment imperative in curriculum renewal. Med Teach. 2018;40(5):443–48.

9. Mirzazadeh A, Gandomkar R, Hejri SM, Hassanzadeh G, Koochak HE, Golestani A, Jafarian A, Jalili M, Nayeri F, Saleh N, Shahi F, Razavi SHE. Undergraduate medical education programme renewal: A longitudinal context, input, process and product evaluation study. Perspect Med Educ. 2016;5:15–23.

10. Aziz S, Mahmood M, Rehman Z. Implementation of CIPP model for quality evaluation at school level: A case study. J Educ Dev. 2018;5(1):189–206. Available from: http://files.eric.ed.gov/fulltext/EJ1180614.pdf

11. Vermont Agency of Education. Plan-do-study-act toolkit: A resource for schools entering the testing phase of the continuous improvement process; 2019. Available from: https://education.vermont.gov/documents/education-quality-assurance-pdsa-toolkit

12. Declaration of Alma-Ata. 1978. Available from: https://www.who.int/publications/almaata_declaration_en.pdf?ua=1

13. Astana Declaration. 2018. Available from: https://www.who.int/docs/default-source/primary-health/declaration/gcphc-declaration.pdf

14. McDonald A, Nettleton J. The KAMFAM study: What the development of a medical student rotation has taught us about the future of family medicine in Malawi [Powerpoint slides]. Available from: https://resourcelibrary.stfm.org/viewdocument/the-kamfam-study-assessing-knowled?CommunityKey=2751b51d-483f-45e2-81de-4faced0a290a&tab=librarydocuments

15. Kassebaum DG, Haynes RA. Relationship between third-year clerkships in family medicine and graduating students' choices of family practice careers. Acad Med. 1992;67(3):217–9.

32

Evidence-based practice

Medical education research

Eliot Rees and Samar Abdelazim Ahmed

SUMMARY OF KEY LEARNING POINTS

- Medical education research is essential to build an evidence base and understand how to select, teach, and assess our future clinicians.
- Research prospectively asks and answers questions to build and test theory. It is distinct from evaluation which retrospectively determines the value of education.
- Medical education research is an enjoyable and rewarding process, especially if built into current educational work, e.g. a new curriculum or teaching tool.
- Relevance, originality, and rigour are fundamental to good research which should aim to generate new knowledge relevant to other educators in different contexts.
- Time and reflection with a mentor are needed to frame research questions before carefully selecting methodology and tools which align well with anticipated answers.
- Different research approaches, post-positivist and constructive, can determine whether to use quantitative, qualitative, or mixed methodology.
- Aim to publish in an appropriate medical education journal making sure you have ethical approval in place.

Introduction

Evidence-based medicine is the cornerstone of clinical practice. It is only through rigorous observation and research that we came to understand that bed rest is not the best treatment for heart attacks and that giving corticosteroids to premature babies increased survival rates. Similarly, it is only through research in medical education that we can know how best to select, train, assess, and support our learners. This chapter aims to introduce you to medical education research, explain why it is important, and point you in the right direction for getting started.

DOI: 10.1201/9781003325734-38

What is research?

Research is the "systematic investigation or inquiry aimed at contributing to knowledge of a theory, topic, etc., by careful consideration, observation, or study of a subject".[1] In many ways, research may be viewed as similar to evaluation as the same methodologies and tools can be used (Chapter 31). The key difference is that research aims to ask and answer questions to generate new knowledge. Evaluation aims to assess the worth of something, such as a teaching programme, which has been already carried out.

> Research aims to build or test theory and draw generalisable findings, whereas evaluation aims to determine the value of an intervention or a programme.

Who needs research?

Simply put, everyone does. All involved in FM education need to engage with research in one way or another. For some, as consumers of research, using the findings from studies to understand how best to design and deliver their educational programmes. For others, as producers of research, undertaking research to address gaps in the literature and increase our collective understanding of FM education. Others will act as reviewers of research; peer reviewing or editing for journals, or as judges on grant committees or for public organisations. These roles are not mutually exclusive, rather they may present a gradual increase in expertise and engagement with research activities.

This chapter is aimed at those who want to start to produce research. If you are responsible for the design or delivery of a FM curriculum, or exploring innovative approaches to teaching, this is an excellent opportunity to research your educational practice and add to the evidence base.

Why produce research?

There are many reasons why one might decide to produce research. It may be that you are curious about an educational issue and want to understand it better. You may aim to develop new skills or feel the need to produce research for your career development. Alternatively, it is a powerful way to prove the worth of, or defend, an educational programme you are involved in. Whatever the reason, conducting research can be interesting, enjoyable, and rewarding.

However, it can be challenging, arduous, and time consuming. Before you set out it is worth considering if you have the time and resources available to commit. Perhaps the most important resource is the support of a research team or mentor. Reach out to those able to support your research endeavours.

Identifying a topic to research

The first and most important step is deciding on a topic to research. If you are going to spend months or years on a research study, it is imperative to choose an area that interests you and will motivate successful completion. There are many sources of potential topics and questions to ask of our current approaches to teaching and learning. Indeed, the very title of this book on "How to integrate FM into the undergraduate curriculum" lends itself to many!

A good way to start is to consider the problems or challenges you encounter routinely in your educational practice. For example, you might find a particular learning approach you have read about does not seem to work in your context in the same way. This could be an area ripe for research. Alternatively, you might find that discussions with colleagues lead to identifying a problem that you could address through research. If you are involved in the design of a new FM curriculum, this is an excellent opportunity to research aspects of the curriculum as it is introduced to improve our collective understanding of how best to support learning in primary care.

> Pick a topic that is going to sustain your enthusiasm and motivate you to complete. Seek the support of an experienced mentor with a shared interest.

Constructing a research question

Having identified a topic to research, then formulate a researchable question. To do this, you first need to explore and understand what is already known about the topic. Conduct a preliminary literature search and see what others have written. This will help you identify what remaining gaps there are in the literature that your study could seek to address. It may well be that your question has already been answered, but the existing literature may help you to refine your question and find a new specific focus.

> Make sure your research study will generate new knowledge or add debate to solve a problem which is relevant to current medical educators and generalisable to their context.

Lingard describes the *problem/gap/hook* heuristic for academic writing.[2] It is useful to start to formulate this early in the design of your study to ensure you are addressing a *problem* where there is a *gap* in the literature which the academic community can see, i.e. *hook*, to their own situation. Conversations with mentors or medical education researchers can be really helpful to point you in the right direction and guide you to frame a question which is focused enough to be achievable.

Once you have identified the problem your research will address and have confirmed there is indeed a gap in the literature, you can begin to craft a research question. There are three essential features of good research questions; relevance, originality, and rigour[3] (Box 32.1).

BOX 32.1 THREE IMPORTANT ELEMENTS OF RESEARCH QUESTION DEVELOPMENT

Relevance	The answer is important to the appropriate stakeholders (teachers, learners, patients)
Originality	The question generates new knowledge and addresses a gap in the published literature. Which debate does it add to?
Rigour	The question is aligned with the methods. Do the research tools generate appropriate data to answer the question?

It is rare that you will find a topic that has not been researched to some extent. If you do, this should ring alarm bells—either you have missed the existing literature or it is a topic of little interest.

There are three scenarios which justify the validity of your research question:

i. When there is a gap in the literature
ii. When the existing research offers conflicting findings
iii. When using a different methodological or theoretical approach generates new insights

It can often be tempting to try to ask a broad question. This is unlikely, however, to provide a meaningful answer in the scope of a small research project. It is far better to hone your question to be more specifically focused and to do something small well rather than something large poorly.

Start with a small, achievable, but well-executed study. Keep it simple. You can always build on it with further research.

Norman offers 12 tips on how to avoid getting your paper rejected.[4] However, if you start considering this at the time of submitting the paper, it is far too late. These should be considered when formulating your research question and designing your study. The most pertinent pitfalls to avoid at the design stage are presented in Box 32.2.

BOX 32.2 TIPS TO CONSIDER WHEN DESIGNING RESEARCH STUDIES

- Avoid, unless theoretically outcomes might differ, applying previous research from one context to another geographical or speciality area; e.g. e-Learning in cardiology is probably as effective as e-Learning in respiratory medicine.

- Avoid comparing a teaching programme or intervention with a "no teaching" control group. Teaching will inevitably be superior to no teaching. A better research design is comparing different teaching approaches to see which is superior.

- Avoid designs that carry unethical educational behaviour where you deprive a group of students of teaching just to create a control group.

- Avoid simplistic evaluations, e.g. student satisfaction or self-reported change in confidence or knowledge. Without objective outcomes, e.g. learning or behaviour change, the use is limited. Best to clarify how or why programmes are successful.

- Avoid research which is only applicable to your organisation. While rigorous evaluation informs local practice, it is rarely of interest to others. Designing research that is generalisable or transferable to other contexts is important.

Approaches to research

Once you have a research question, you need to design and operationalise a study that will enable you to find the answer. In clinical research, the hierarchy of evidence dictates that systematic reviews and meta-analyses of randomised control trials are the highest-quality design. In contrast, in medical education research, different methodological approaches are valued equally. What is most important is that the methodology and tools are well-aligned to your research question. This is called internal coherence.[5]

First, consider which research paradigm is most appropriate for your question. There are several paradigms, but for the purposes of simplicity, we will discuss the two most used in medical education research: post-positivism and constructivism (Table 32.1). For a fuller discussion of paradigms, see Brown and Dueñas.[6]

TABLE 32.1 An overview of post-positivist and constructivist research paradigms

Paradigm	Post-positivism	Constructivism
Ontology (The nature of reality)	There is a single objective reality that researchers need to discover	There are multiple, potentially competing, realities that are constructed by individuals
Epistemology (How we can come to know about reality)	Knowledge can be generated through objective, reliable, and valid measurements. It is important to recognise bias and how that may affect knowledge generated.	Knowledge is subjective. It depends on the researcher and the researched interactions
Methodology (Research approach)	Usually quantitative	Usually qualitative
Example methods (The specific tools)	Surveys, assessments, experiments, big data	Interviews, focus groups, observation, documents

In post-positivist research, researchers believe there is a single true answer to their question, and their job is to collect objective data without influence from the researcher. This research typically involves quantitative methods and seeks to test hypotheses which may be generated from existing theories.

Constructivist researchers, on the other hand, believe that reality is socially constructed and therefore there will be multiple and sometimes conflicting realities experienced by different individuals. The researcher's job is to collect data that will enable them to better understand how these realities are experienced. This typically involves qualitative methods and a recognition that understanding is generated through the interactions between the researchers and participants. Constructivist research does not aim to test hypotheses but may be useful in developing or refining theory.

Based on your research question, you may find that one is more appropriate than the other. Consider, for example, the following two research questions:

1. Does duration of FM placement during medical school influence learners' aspirations to become family physicians?
2. What do students value in longitudinal FM rotations?

The first question implies a clear hypothesis to be tested. As such, this question would lend itself better to a post-positivist study using quantitative methods. The second question, however, does not have a clear hypothesis. This question may be more suitable for an exploratory constructivist study using qualitative methods. Often it can be useful to use both approaches to investigate the same topic in turn. For example, you might conduct an exploratory constructivist study that generates theory which you then test in a post-positivist quantitative study. Through doing so, you can start to build a programme of research.

> Think about what approach is most suitable after you have agreed on the research question. It is easier then to make sure the methodology aligns with and can answer it.

It is worth noting that not all research has to collect primary data. Often an evidence synthesis can be a useful starting point to formally describe the current state of knowledge regarding a specific topic. For further details on specific research methods for primary care educational research, see "How to Do Primary Care Educational Research: A Practical Guide".[7]

Ethical approval

When planning your study, it is imperative that you submit your plan for review by an ethics committee. Any research containing data from human participants requires review by an ethics committee. Most journals will now not accept papers for publication without confirmation of ethical approval.[8] Some authors argue that their papers are evaluation studies, but it is better to have obtained confirmation of exemption from the chair of an ethics committee.

Dissemination

Once you have finished your research, it is time to share your findings. Presenting at meetings and conferences can be a useful way to communicate your learning and stimulate discussion with others with shared interests. It is also a good way of building your professional network.

We encourage you to consider how you will share your findings right from the start of your project. In fact, recent research has shown that authors that choose a target journal early in the research process are more likely to have their papers accepted by their first-choice journal.[9] While there are many factors to consider when choosing a journal, thinking about which one will enable your work to be seen by the right audience is a good place to start.[9]

Conclusion

This chapter has introduced you to the value of medical education research and discussed how to go about identifying a problem worth researching and constructing a research question. Researching your FM curricular innovations and disseminating your findings may help add useful knowledge to the field and will develop your professional profile.

References

1. "Research, n.1." OED Online, Oxford University Press. June 2022. Available from: www. oed.com/view/Entry/163432 (Accessed 30 July 2022).
2. Lingard L. Joining a conversation: The problem/gap/hook heuristic. Perspect Med Educ. 2015;4(5):252–53. doi: 10.1007/s40037-015-0211-y.
3. Mattick K, Johnston J, de la Croix A. How to write a good research question. Clin Teach. 2018;15:104–08. doi: 10.1111/tct.12776
4. Norman G. Data dredging, salami-slicing, and other successful strategies to ensure rejection: Twelve tips on how to not get your paper published. Adv Health Sci Educ. 2014;19:1–5. doi: 10.1007/s10459-014-9494-8
5. Palermo C, Reidlinger DP, Rees CE. Internal coherence matters: Lessons for nutrition and dietetics research. Nutr Diet. 2021;78(3):252–67. doi: 10.1111/1747-0080.12680.
6. Brown MEL, Dueñas AN. A medical science Educator's guide to selecting a research paradigm: Building a basis for better research. Med Sci Educ. 2019;30(1):545–53. doi: 10.1007/s40670-019-00898-9.
7. Akman M, Wass V, Goodyear-Smith F. How to do primary care educational research: A practical guide. CRC Press; 2021.
8. Thistlethwaite J, Trumble S. Ethics, publication and the clinical teacher. Clin Teach. 2012;9:353–55.
9. Rees EL, Burton O, Asif A, Eva KW. A method for the madness: An international survey of health professions education authors' journal choice. Perspect Med Educ. 2022;11(3):165–72. doi: 10.1007/s40037-022-00698-9.

Faculty development and continuous professional development

Laura Goldman and Nguyễn Minh Tam

SUMMARY OF KEY LEARNING POINTS

- Faculty development (FD) increases faculty confidence, satisfaction, motivation, effectiveness, academic output, and career advancement.
- Community-based tutors are essential to family medicine (FM) undergraduate education. Understanding their motivations to teach and the challenges they face is important.
- Developing a FD programme for community tutors involves conducting a needs assessment, setting goals, developing an implementation plan, and conducting an evaluation.
- An effective programme includes a defined strategy, experiential learning, community-building, longitudinal design, institutional support, and flexibility to adapt to changing needs.
- Evaluation of an FD programme's impact on participants is best achieved by a triangulation of methods aiming to understand the sustained impact on learning and behaviour change.
- FD is essential to building an FM academic department able to accomplish teaching, research, and clinical care goals.

Background

FD is defined as any activity that is undertaken to improve the knowledge, skill, and behaviours of faculty as teachers, educators, leaders, managers, researchers, and scholars. In the past two decades, FD programmes have been utilised by most medical schools to improve teaching and learning effectiveness and to promote career advancement for faculty.

The literature has highlighted the benefits of FD programmes to individual teachers. Most studies have found overall high satisfaction. Self-reported gains in knowledge of educational principles and of skills in specific teaching strategies

DOI: 10.1201/9781003325734-39

result in increased confidence, enthusiasm, and a more positive attitude towards teaching. In addition to increased effectiveness in the classroom or clinical setting, observed changes include new educational courses, leadership positions, increased academic output, and career advancement. Less is known about the effect of FD programmes on student behaviour or organisational change, but some programmes report improved networks of support for teaching among colleagues.[1]

> FD programmes result in increased tutor knowledge, ability, confidence, and motivation to teach. This can enhance educational change, academic output, and career progression.

Community-based learning is a key feature of FM training. A challenge in most settings is recruiting and retaining community tutors. Many teachers volunteer their time because of intrinsic rewards linked to the joy of teaching, value in passing on knowledge, and opportunity to shape the careers of future physicians. Barriers include time constraints, productivity demands, institutional bureaucracy, negative teaching experiences and electronic health records. Targeted FD programmes that address tutor needs, such as teaching with the patient present, integrating students into the office, and giving feedback to challenging students, can increase teaching competence and confidence. This has been linked to increased motivation to teach.[2,3]

Developing a faculty development programme for community tutors

Developing a FD programme for community tutors should be based on local needs. Box 33.1 outlines the steps to take to achieve this.

Developing an FD programme involves three steps: planning, implementation, and evaluation. The planning stage involves a needs assessment and defining goals and measurable outcomes.[4]

BOX 33.1 STEPS TO DEVELOP A FACULTY DEVELOPMENT PROGRAMME FOR COMMUNITY TUTORS

1. Conduct a needs assessments to fit local context through site visits, surveys, tutor self-report, and/or evaluations by students and peers.
2. Based on assessment, FD programmes can be developed on different levels: Individual tutor, learning process, or educational outcome.
3. Teaching competencies for clinical tutors can be used to develop programme goals.
4. Develop an implementation plan that includes content, educational strategy, and logistics for delivery of the programme.
5. Most FD programme evaluations rely on self-reported satisfaction. A triangulation of evaluations that include self-report, peers, and students is the most reliable method.

Needs assessment, goals, and outcomes

FD courses vary in content and formats. There is no clear evidence supporting any one approach. Needs assessments to design FD programmes to fit the local context are often achieved through site visits, surveys, and evaluations by students, peers, and tutor self-report. A survey of 112 (of 141 total) FM clerkship directors in the United States and Canada found that informal conversations with tutors (76%) and teaching evaluations by students (61%) were most often used to determine FD needs.[5] Surveys of medical educators in India, Singapore, and China have been used to target FD efforts.[6]

Results of needs assessment may lead to FD programmes on several levels. These include individual tutor competencies in terms of knowledge, skills, and behaviour; learning process such as small group or clinical teaching; or educational outcomes, such as better student assessment, the use of Objective Structured Clinical Examinations (OSCEs), measuring professionalism, or research.[6]

> Recruiting and retaining FM community tutors requires an understanding of the local context and their personal expectations and motivations to teach and any barriers to volunteering.

Teaching competencies for community tutors with well-defined performance indicators can be used to develop goals and outcomes. Brink et al.[7] identified 5 competency domains and 21 teaching competencies specific to medical student community tutors in FM. For example, in the domain of learner centredness, competencies include preparing the environment for the learner, orienting the learner, ascertaining the learner's knowledge and skills, responding to learner's cultural context, and helping learners develop learning goals aligned to patient needs.

Bartlett et al.[8] reported on 41 studies from around the world that measured health professional tutor competence. They identified 17 evidence-based competencies, of which 11 had performance indicators. Examples include demonstrating respect for learners and commitment to excellence in teaching.[8] Assessments of tutors by peers, students, and self-report using these performance indicators can be employed to identify deficiencies. Thus, FD programmes can be targeted to modifiable behaviours. Qualities of effective community tutors for preclinical students include provision of adequate orientation to the clinic, student independence in patient assessment, and time devoted to teaching and giving feedback.[9]

> Evidence-based performance indicators of health professional teaching competencies can be used to assess and give feedback on modifiable behaviours.

Implementation

After the FD programme goals have been determined, the next step is deciding how to deliver the programme in terms of content, educational strategy, and logistics.

Content

Sorinola and Thistlethwaite[10] conducted a literature review of global FD activities in FM. The majority of FD programmes focus on teaching instructional topics, such as concepts in adult education, writing objectives, teaching methods, assessment, and feedback. Communication skills and professional topics such as mentoring, portfolios, programme evaluation, and leadership are commonly included. Research, technology, and organisational skills are less frequently offered.

Educational strategy

Adult learning, experiential learning, and learner-centred approaches are the three most used educational strategies, although only 25% of programmes are grounded in a conceptual framework[10] (Chapter 19).

FD is commonly delivered as short courses, seminars, or workshops. Longitudinal programmes can lead to an award or certification if, over 1–2 years, a faculty member devotes a certain amount of time on a regular basis to acquire knowledge and/or skills. Instructional techniques are almost always experiential, and include small group discussions, interactive exercises, role plays, simulation, videotape review, case-based workshops, peer coaching, web-based learning, and mentoring.[10]

> FD is best based on adult self-directed experiential learning in short courses or workshops based on interactive exercises. Regular involvement can result in awards and certification.

The most common types of FD for undergraduate community tutors in the United States and Canada are personalised feedback based on student evaluations (71%), site visits (61%), and face-to- face tutor development sessions (52%). Also frequently employed are online educational curricula (44%), targeted articles or clinical teaching (23%), and pocket cards (21%).[5]

Logistics

Barriers to FD for community tutors need to be addressed before implementation. The most challenging are tutor time availability, geographical distribution of tutors, financial resources, clerkship director time, and competition from other programmes.

Creative methods to overcome these barriers include using listservs, online discussion modules, podcasts, and online resources for teaching physicians.[3,5]

An example of an online resource is Teaching Physician, https://www.teaching-physician.org, a website maintained by the Society for Teachers in FM. This subscription service is a comprehensive web-based resource that connects medical schools to community tutors. It provides point-of-need instruction with videos, tips, and links to in-depth information on a long list of tutoring topics. Sections on preparation, tutoring principles, what to teach, teaching strategies, feedback, evaluation, etc. can be easily accessed by tutors depending on interest.

Evaluation

Most evaluations of FD programmes in FM rely on self-reported satisfaction surveys. Rated most highly are interactive exercises, experiential practice, small group discussions, and the ability to become part of a community of scholars. Participants report positive changes in confidence and comfort in teaching and giving feedback. A few studies report higher level changes, including behavioural or organisational change. In these studies, outcomes were generally positive and included increased use of new teaching techniques, better communication, increased scholarly activity, new curriculum, leadership, and faculty retention. A triangulation of evaluations of the participant, which includes self-report, peers' and learners' feedback is the most reliable method.[10]

> Evaluation of FD programmes should aim to look beyond satisfaction to explore behavioural or organisational change. Triangulation of methods is best for appraising tutors.

Key features of successful FD initiatives in family medicine

Components of effective FD have been outlined in the literature. These include evidenced-based instructional design, relevant content, experiential learning, and opportunities for practice, feedback, and reflection. Highly valued is longitudinal programme design, educational projects that allow for application of learning in the workplace, intentional community-building, and institutional support.[1]

FM presents unique challenges for FD. Training must be adapted to the participant's unique home practice environment, so that lessons learned can be applied to the workplace. Programmes must be flexible and quickly adaptable to respond to changing needs. The COVID-19 pandemic is an example of the critical importance of delivering content rapidly. Programmes must be evaluated for quality improvement purposes, and funding and protected time for participants is critical to success whenever possible.[10]

Box 33.2 outlines how FD can be used to build an academic FM department.

BOX 33.2 BUILDING AN ACADEMIC FM DEPARTMENT
THROUGH FACULTY DEVELOPMENT

1. Local faculty should be aggressively recruited for advanced training in FM.
2. Multi-institutional collaborations within country enable sharing of resources and experience, provide support, and allow dissemination of accomplishments.
3. Non-FM specialists can be used initially to expand the pool of trainers.
4. Short-term FD programmes abroad can be used to scale up faculty.
5. Local FD programmes and advance degree training should be developed for sustainability.
6. FD opportunities should be strategically allocated to increase capacity depending on department needs.
7. Masters and PhD projects should be integrated into department goals.

Building an academic FM department through faculty development in a low-resource country

Our discussion has focused on FD for community tutors. However, FD has a critical role in building an FM department in a medical school to meet core functions that include education, research, and patient care (Chapter 5).

The Hue University of Medicine and Pharmacy (UMP) in Vietnam presents a case study in building an academic department in a low-resource country with no prior FM experience. In an effort to strengthen the primary health care system, the Ministry of Health sponsored the "Extending Improvements in the Primary Care System through Expansion of Medical Education & System Supports in Vietnam" project from 2013 to 2016. FD was a core component of this multi-institutional collaboration that included three public universities in Vietnam and Boston University Family Medicine.[11,12]

Collaborative Centers of Excellence were established, and faculty were recruited for advanced degree training both within and outside Vietnam. Leaders and non-FM specialist faculty were enrolled in longitudinal and short-term fellowships at Boston University. A new Masters in FM Programme was established at Hanoi UMP. Despite multiple challenges, the masters programme gained permanent government approval ensuring sustainability.

FD is important when creating academic FM departments. Longitudinal collaborations with government, international institutions, and recruiting non-FM experts can build sustainability.

Training local field trainers in teaching methods proved to be more challenging than anticipated, and output was limited. This was attributed to too few core faculty to meet the extra time demands to train field trainers. Faculty did receive some local university training that included working clinically alongside specialists, and various courses in teaching.

Hue UMP also has a longitudinal collaboration with the University of Gent in Belgium to train Hue faculty as PhDs in FM. Strategically enrolling PhD students on a gradual basis has enabled the FM department to identify internal needs, support scholars, and strengthen research and education capacity. In 2022, one PhD has been granted and three others are in the programme.

A high internal synergy has been created through this project with complementary activities, such as curriculum revision, production of textbooks, e-learning modules, development of trainings and guidelines, and PhD–research. All these activities have been strongly linked to building up capacity and outreach on FM.

Hue UMP has become a flagship centre for FM in Vietnam. One collateral result has been the establishment of a new formal educational infrastructure for the specialty of FM during medical school and postgraduate training across all of Vietnam. A future goal is to develop a FM PhD programme in Vietnam at Hue UMP. Box 33.2 summarises the lessons learnt from this project.

References

1. Steinert Y, Mann K, Anderson B, Barnett BM, Centeno A, Naismith L et al. A systematic review of faculty development initiatives designed to enhance teaching effectiveness: A 10-year update: BEME Guide no. 40. Med Teach. 2016;38 (8):769–86. doi: 10.1080/0142159X.2016.1181851

2. Minor S, Huffman M, Lewis P, Kost A, Prunuske J. Community tutor perspectives on recruitment and retention: The CoPPRR study. Fam Med. 2019;51(5):389–98. doi: 10.22454/FamMed.2019.937544

3. Christner JG, Dallaghan GB, Briscoe G, Casey P, Fincher RME, Manfred LM et al. The community tutor crisis: Recruiting and retaining community-based faculty to teach medical students—A shared perspective from the alliance for clinical education. Teach Learn Med. 2016;28 (3):329–36. doi: 10.1080/10401334.2016.1152899

4. McLean M, Cilliers F, Van Wyk J. Faculty development: Yesterday, today and tomorrow. Med Teach. 2008;30(6):555–84. doi: 10.1080/01421590802109834

5. Drowos J, Baker S, Harrison SL, Minor S, Chessman AW, Baker D. Faculty development for medical school community-based faculty: A Council of Academic Family Medicine Educational Research Alliance study exploring institutional requirements and challenges. Acad Med. 2017;92(8):1175–80. doi: 10.1097/ACM.0000000000001626

6. Johnson B, Cayley WE, Nguyen BM, Larson P, Colon-Gonzalez M, del C, Christine Gibson C, Evensen A. Faculty development in family medicine education: What is needed? Pan Afr Med J. 2017;26:1–4. doi: 10.11604/pamj.2017.26.141.9069

7. Brink D, Simpson D, Crouse B, Morzinski J, Bower R, Westra D. Teaching competencies for community tutors. Fam Med. 2018;50(5):359–63. doi: 10.22454/FamMed.2018.578747

8. Bartlett AD, Um IS, Luca EJ, Krass I, Carl R, Schneider CR. Measuring and assessing the competencies of tutors in health professions: A systematic scoping review. BMC Med Educ. 2020;20(1):1–9. doi: 10.1186/s12909-020-02082-9

9. Lie D, Boker J, Dow ED, Murata P, Encinas J, Gutierrez JD, Morrison EH. Attributes of effective community tutors for pre-clerkship medical students. Med Teach. 2009;31(3):251–59. doi: 10.1080/01421590802139765

10. Sorinol OO, Thistlethwaite J. A systematic review of faculty development activities in family medicine. Med Teach. 2013;35(7). doi: 10.3109/0142159X.2013.770132

11. Montegut AJ, Cartwright CA, Schirmer JM, Cummings S. An international consultation: The development of family medicine in Vietnam. Fam Med. 2004;36(5):352–56.

12. Montegut AJ, Schirmer J, Cartwright C, Holt C, Chuc NTK, An PN, Cummings S. Creation of postgraduate training programs for family medicine in Vietnam. Fam Med. 2007;39(9):634–38.

Index

Note: Locators in *italics* represent figures and **bold** indicate tables in the text.

A

Academic leadership, 36
Academic primary care, 35–41
Academy of Family Physicians of India
  (AFPI), 31
Accreditation Council for Graduate
  Medical Education (ACGME), 77,
  180, 199
Advocacy, 95, 143
Agenda-led Outcome-based Analysis
  (ALOBA), 222, 223
Annals of Internal Medicine, 196
Apprenticeship learning, 122–123
  benefits of, 123–124
  challenges of, 124–125, **125**
  cognitive, 125–126
  solutions in, **125**
  student participation in, 127
Apprenticeship model, 123, 126, 206
Asian medical schools, 55–57
Assessing clinical competency, 215–216
Assessment, 229
  acceptability, 230
  case-based discussions, 232
  comprehensive competency-based, 215
  concepts in, 229–230
  cost, 230
  cultures, 189
  direct observation, 234
  educational impact, 230
  feasibility, 230
  FM doctors in, 235
  formative, 213, 216, 217, 230
  long cases, 233
  oral examinations, 232
  portfolios, 234–235
  programmatic, *218*
  reliability, 229
  short answer questions (SAQs), 232
  short cases, 233
  single best answer (SBA), 231
  summative, 213, 216, 217, 230
  supervisor's report, 234
  360-degree feedback, 234
  tools for, 229
  validity, 230
Astana Declaration of 2018, 15, 44, 84

B

Balint, Michael, 53
Bandura's social cognitive learning
    theory, 150
Barbezat, D.P., 199
Barnett, R., 197
Barriers
  for change, 45
  potential, 44
Bartlett, A.D., 264
Bates, J., 132
Behavioural deficits, 241

Bhise, V., 187
Blended learning (BL), 155–161
  asynchronous, 155–156
  benefits of, 157–158
  blended block, 157
  blended presentation and
    interaction, 156
  challenges of, 158–159
  COVID-19, 160–161
  fully online, 157
  models of, **157**
  online and, 156
  synchronous, 155
  tips, 159–160
  types of, 156–157
Boehler, M.L., 224
Brink, D., 264
Burgess, A., 182, 183
Burnout, 196
Bush, M., 199

C
Calgary Cambridge framework, 176, *177*
Canadian Interprofessional Health
  Collaborative framework, 138
Case-based discussions, 232
Chen, H.C., 153
Classroom learning, 117–118
Clinical and procedural skills, 179–180
  assess, 183–184
  teach, 180–181
Clinical courage, 191–192
Clinical placements, 116
Clinical reasoning
  application of, 165–166
  definitions of, 164
  development techniques, 166–168
Cloning model, 206
Coaching, 203
Collaborative Centers of Excellence, 267
Collaborative practice, 138–139
College of Family Physicians of Canada
  (CFPC), 12
Communication skills
  cultural influence, 176–177
  discuss stage, 173–174
  greet stage, 172
  invite stage, 172–173
  multimorbidity, 175
  therapeutic relationship, 174–175
  uncertainty, 175–176

Community-based curriculum, 63
Community-based learning, 263
Community-based primary healthcare
  centres, 66
Community-based training (CBT), 215
Community-oriented primary care
  (COPC), 62
Comorbidity, 38
Competency, 213, 216, 231
Competency-based curriculum, 77–79
  characteristics of, 78
  operationalising a family medicine, 81
Competency-based education (CBE),
  76–77
Competency-based medical education
  (CBME), 213–215
Complexity, 189–190
Conducting programme evaluation,
  249–251
Consortium of Longitudinal Integrated
  Clerkship (CLIC), 131
Context-input-process-product
  (CIPP), 251
Continuity principles, 131
COVID-19, 160–161
  pandemic, 6, 49, 192, 196, 198, 266
Critical reflection, 97
Cultural humility, 150–151
Cultural influence, 176–177
Curriculum, 48
  formal, 98–99
  hidden, 101–102
  informal, 100–101

D
Danczak, A., 187
Decision-making, 73–74
Direct observation of procedural skills
  (DOPS), 232
Disease, 71–72
Dissemination, 261

E
Educational programmes, 241
Ellaway, R.H., 132
Elwyn, G., 73
Enid, Michael, 53
Entrustable professional activities
  (EPAs), 77, 218
Ethical approval, 260
Evidence-based practice, 255

Experiential learning, 147–154
  active participation, 151–153
  cultural humility, 150–151
  encourage reflective practice, 148–150
  Kolb's cycle, *148*
  Kolb's experiential learning theory, 148
"Exploratory Model Approach," 151

F
Faculty
  responsive, 67
  training, 120
Faculty development (FD) programme,
    64–65, 78, 262–263
  assessments, 264
  for community tutors, 263
  content, 265
  educational strategy, 265
  evaluations of, 266
  implementation, 265
  logistics, 265–266
  low-resource country, 267–268
Family
  definition of, 73
  participation, 74
  physician as a role model, 90–91
  physicians, 182, 203
  placements, 73
  role of, 73
Family medicine (FM)
  advocacy in, 143
  alignment of assessment with, 214–215
  characteristics of, **79**
  clerkships, 252
  clinical exposure, 119
  countries, 31–32
  definition of, 13–14
  doctor, 94, 229
  early exposure to, 115–120
  educators, 117
  faculty, 47, 117
  faculty and the students, 49–50
  faculty members, 200
  global challenges, 12–13
  growth of, 32
  health systems, 15
  humanism in, 52–57
  implementation of, 43
  importance of, 44–45
  leadership in, 143
  in medical schools, 30–31

  nurturing humanism in, 54–55
  principles of, 11–12, 119
  role in society, 15
  role modelling, 14–15
  terminology, 11
  training, 30
  value of, 79–81
  values–based recruitment, 112–113
Family practice
  hidden curriculum in, **102**
  informal curriculum in, **101**
  role models, 100
Farajpour, A., 216
Feedback, 221
  constructive, 217, 230–231
  formulae, 222–223
  importance of observation, 222
  problems with, 223–226
  360-degree, 234
  tips, 226–227
Flexner, Abraham, 115
Flexner model, 70
FM placements
  active learning in, 126–127
  cognitive apprenticeship learning in,
    125–126
  role modelling, 127–128
Formal curriculum, 98–99

G
Garcia-Rodriguez, J.A., 183
Garrison, D.R., 156
Generalism, 3–4, 39, 79–81
  challenges of, 6–7
  evolution of, 5
  and family medicine, 5
  framework, *4*
  necessary, 6
  principles, 79, **80**
Gibbs reflective cycle, 148, *149*
Global differences, 204
Globalisation, 55
Graham, C.R., 156

H
Hauer, K. E., 132
Health, 71–72
  systems, 46
Healthcare, 3–8
  professionals, 116
Hege, I., 156

Hidden curriculum, 101–102
Hippocrates, 5
Hirsh, D., 131
Horizontal integration, 87
Houghton, A., 197
Hue University of Medicine and
    Pharmacy (UMP), 267, 268
Humanisation, 118–119
Humanism, 52–53
  Asian medical schools, 55–57
  in family medicine, 54–55
  habits of, 55
  humanistic healthcare professional, **53**
  important, 54
  undergraduate curriculum, 54

I
Illness, 71–72
Indicators of Social Accountability Tool
    (ISAT), 21
Informal curriculum, 100–101
Integrated curriculum
  benefits of, 89
  generalist learning outcomes, 85–86
  horizontal, 87
  SPICES model, 86
  spiral curriculum, 88–89
  vertical, 87
Interpreter, 165
Interprofessional learning (IPL), 137–138
  approaches to, 139–140
  challenges to, 138–139
  change management, 142
  domains, **139**
  implementation of, 140, **141**

K
Kanuka, H., 156
Kirkpatrick, D., 142
Kleinman, Arthur, 172
Knowledge, democratisation of, 93
Kolb, D.A., 140
Konkin, J., 192
Kouzes, J.M., 200

L
Lasagna, Louis, 201
Lave, J., 152
Lea, A., 187
Leadership, 143
  literature, 200

Learning environment
  conducive, 225
  importance of, 225–226
Lingard, L., 257
Longitudinal integrated clerkships
    (LIC), 130–132
  categories of, 131
  communities, 134
  development of, 133
  enablers and challenges, 133–134
  establishing an, 133
  rural, 132
Lower middle-income country (LMIC),
    90, 132

M
Marks, N., 197
McWhinney, Ian, 11, 14
Medical care
  ecology of, 37, 116
  humanisation of, 118–119
Medical education
  challenge of changing traditional, 85
  community-based, 64
  evolution of, 201
  leaders, 66
  role of, 7–8
Medical school
  assessments, 213
  curriculum, 48, 181
  early FM exposure in, 119–120
  high-quality research, 108
  scrutiny of, 107
  selection, 108–110
  tools, **111**
Medical students
  issues, 238
  knowledge, 238–240
  skill deficits, 238–240
  socialisation of, 117
Medical student struggles
  factors, **239**
  importance of, 237–238
  institutional requirements for, **243**
  multifaceted approach, 242–243
  nature of, 238
  personal and health issues, 241–242
Mentorship, 202
  apprenticeship model, 206
  attributes, 208
  benefits of, 207–209, **208**

cloning model, 206
  effective, 209
  feedback, 217
  formal, 206
  informal, 206
  instrumental, 206
  nurturing model, 206–207
  roles, 202
Michels, M.E.J., 180, 182
Miller, G.E., 231
Miller's pyramid, 216, *231*
Mini-clinical evaluation exercise
  (mini-CEX), 232
Morgan, H., 197
Multi-mini interviews (MMIs), 111–112
Multimorbidity, 175, 189

N
1978 WHO Alma Ata Declaration, 15
Nurturing model, 206–207

O
Objective structured clinical
  examination (OSCE), 217, 233
Oral examinations, 232

P
Patient-centred care, 70
Patient-centred clinical method,
  70–71, *71*
Patterson, F., 110
Peabody, Francis, 54
Pendleton's model, 223
Plan-do-study-act (PDSA), 252
Population needs
  assessment, 64
  based curricula, 63
  core elements, 65
  of country, 61–62
  into the curriculum, 66
  identify, 62
Portfolios, 234–235
Posner, B., 200
Primary care (PC), 28, *29*
  community-oriented, 62–63
  comorbidity, 38
  paradox of, 38
  research networks, 39
  role of, 63
Primary healthcare (PHC) system, 28,
  29, 214

Professionalism, 92–93, 97, 241
  elements of, 95
  nurturing, 94
  teaching, 96–97
Programme evaluation/quality
  improvement (PE/QI), 247
  benefits, 248–249
  cyclic process, *248*
  educators, 248
  institutions, 248
  patients and society, 249
  programme leadership, 248
  students, 248

Q
Quality improvement (QI), 247
  mechanisms for, 251–252

R
Reflection, 149
Reflexivity, 239
Regulation, 64
Remediation, 240, 242–244
Research, 256
  approaches to, 259–260
  constructing a research question,
    257–259
  constructivist, 260
  identifying a topic to, 257
  paradigms, **259**
  post-positivist, 260
Responsive faculty, 67
Risk, 191
Rogers, Carl, 6
R2C2 model, 223

S
Safety netting, 193
Sawyer, T., 183
SBAR communication tool, 168
Self-assessment, 218
Self-regulation, 150, 239
Service learning, 199
Short answer questions (SAQs), 232
Single best answer (SBA), 231
Situational judgement tests (SJTs), 112
Social accountability, 17–25, 184
  adapting, 20–23
  biomedical approach, 19
  definition, 18
  in health professions education, 17

lack of congruency, 19
primary healthcare development, 19
principles, 19–20
terminology, 19
Socialisation, 117
Social network theory, 140
Sorinola, O.O., 265
SPICES model, 86
Spiral curriculum, 88–89
Starfield, Barbara, 6
Steuer, N., 197
Stewart, M., 70
Student engagement, 66, 217–218
Supervision, 203
  assessing activities, 205–206
  directing activities, 205–206
  roles, 203, 205
Supervisor's report, 234

T
Technology, 161
Ten Cate, O., 192
Therapeutic relationship, 174–175
Thistlethwaite, J.A., 265
Traditional biomedical model, 115–116
Training supervisors, 206

U
UK Clinical Reasoning in Medical
  Education (CReME), 166
Uncertainty, 175–176, 187
  challenge and opportunity of,
    186–187
  definition, 187–187
Undifferentiated illness, 189
Universal Health Care (UHC), 27, 32

University of Pretoria's FM Department
  (UPFM), 47

V
Values, 93
Values-based education
  dissensus, 96
  exploring global, 95–96
Values-based practice, 94–95
Values-based practice (VBP), 93, 95, 97
Values-based recruitment (VBR), 112,
  113
Vertical integration, 87

W
Well-being
  be active, 198
  connect, 198
  definition, 196–197
  keep learning, 198–199
  mental, 198
  physical, 198
  problem, 195–196
  in undergraduate education, 197–198
Wenger, E., 152
WONCA, 13–14
Workforce
  healthcare, 27
  primary care, 28–29
  primary healthcare system, 28
  sustainable, 32–33
Workplace-based assessment (WPBA),
  216, 217
World Health Organisation (WHO), 15,
  27, 62, 180–181
Worley, P., 131

Printed in the United States
by Baker & Taylor Publisher Services